TRUST &
BETRAYAL

Morality and the Emotions in Surgery

The prominence of informed consent in contemporary medical practice has created the impression that trusting doctors is somehow a second-best moral option. However, in this richly detailed and highly personal book, David Macintosh demonstrates how trust is, in fact, the essential glue that holds medicine together. Drawing on his extensive experience as a surgeon, Macintosh's candid and insightful investigation into medical trust and betrayal probes deeply into what it means for medical practitioners to be truly worthy of their patients' trust. In doing so, Macintosh lays bare the emotional contours and nuances of the practitioner–patient relationship, and shows us how trust can flourish here, despite the ineliminable uncertainties of medicine.

Justin Oakley, Monash University

TRUST & BETRAYAL

Morality and the Emotions in Surgery

David Macintosh

AUSTRALIAN SCHOLARLY

© David Macintosh 2016

First published 2016 by
Australian Scholarly Publishing Pty Ltd
7 Lt Lothian St North, North Melbourne, Victoria 3051
www.scholarly.info / enquiries@scholarly.info / (61) (3) 93296963

ISBN 978-1-925333-58-9

Cover design by Amelia Walker

Whatever matters to human beings trust is the atmosphere in which it thrives.

Sissela Bok, *Lying*

Now I can ask if you will join your force to mine, and hope to speak freely of many hidden things. There is at my age a question of trust. There is a need to speak my heart, to unlock my locks, to unveil my mysteries. Great things are afoot.

Salman Rushdie, *The Moor's Last Sigh*

Contents

Chapter One: Empathy

It was always very difficult for me to tell someone they were dying. No course or lecture about how to approach it or what words to use seemed to help. I eventually worked out that the actual words I used did not seem to matter. A person always hears the word as meaning or implying 'death', no matter the euphemism. Most helpful was the unspoken communication: a kind voice, a light touch to the arm, eye contact, understanding, empathy, and many other small, sincere things. But nothing can really soften the blow. The worst thing to do is to be evasive. I can remember avoiding a young woman who had suddenly developed secondary tumours in her lungs and I waited until a senior colleague told her. I was ashamed of this. It was my responsibility. I betrayed her trust in me to be there for her, no matter how difficult it would have been for me.[1]

With Alice it was different. I was a little older, a little wiser and much more willing to be involved and to share her vulnerability, yet I still had a long way to go. I wrote a poem as a way to understand my own reactions to her illness and death, and her reaction to me. This happened many years ago and I had almost forgotten about the poem until I was reminded of the importance of poetry in distilling the essence of our emotions and I remembered it and knew where to find it. As I read the poem now I can see faults in the wording and style but I have not altered it, as this is how I felt and expressed myself at the time. It is at the end of this section.

The emotions I had when I told someone they had cancer were very complex. There has been a lot written about power in the doctor–patient relationship, but not so much on how it affects the doctor. Being powerful is seductive and made me feel good about myself. Self-empowerment is one thing, power over others is another. I had knowledge about the patient and the power to decide how to express and use it. On the other hand, I was usually affected by a patient's reaction to me, because it was not possible to avoid empathy and identification with her, not to mention my own projected vulnerability, as I knew that someday her plight could be mine. More importantly, perhaps, I saw myself reflected in Alice's eyes. Did she ever see my own uncertainty and fear, and if she did, did that help or hinder her? How much did her reaction to me affect me and make me more or less useful to her? How much could she trust me to genuinely support and care for her, in spite of my own manifest inadequacies? These questions really motivated me to do my best; as to be trustworthy, to be a good doctor, mattered a lot to me. And I could see how well I was doing by observing Alice's reaction. She helped me understand how she saw me.

In many ways Alice was like most other patients, yet she was also uniquely able to express back to me how she felt about me. I knew she trusted me but I realised she was aware of my human deficiencies and accepted them. To her, perhaps, I was not some powerful being but a fairly normal man trying to do his job. Nevertheless, I think she realised I cared about her and I hope she understood how much she moved and influenced me. Alice was referred to me by her family doctor, who happened to be an old school friend of mine. She had noticed a soft swelling on top of her mid foot that was increasing in size. She was anxious about seeing a surgeon and my friend later ruefully confessed to me that he had tried to reassure her by saying 'don't worry he won't cut your foot off'. The swelling turned out to be an invasive malignant soft tissue tumour that had spread through a number of the small joints in her foot. We consulted various cancer therapists and all agreed the correct treatment was an amputation through the lower leg followed by chemotherapy. Alice accepted this calmly, although admitted to being disturbed when I consulted with a plastic surgeon about the possibility of limb-saving surgery who promptly drew on her leg what he thought were the best lines for my incision.

I felt sad for her and so inept, as I was not able to easily discuss with her what would happen to her and how she felt about it.

Very few people would freely choose to have an amputation, although it is not unheard of. Even patients for whom I have advised amputation of the small toe because of deformity and pain are usually very reluctant to agree to it. I have always disliked doing it as I seem to share some primitive horror of the idea. The severed limb is usually placed in a plastic bag and sent away from the theatre, in Alice's case to the pathologist for further study, before being disposed of according to the processes of the law. It always felt to me we were disposing of the evidence of some horrible crime. I became used to it over the years but the feeling never completely went away. Alice had her amputation and coped with the rigours of chemotherapy. Her husband came with her for her consultations and was always caring and supporting. Everything seemed to be going well. Then one night I was awakened by a telephone call telling me she had been admitted to hospital gasping for breath due to the presence of multiple secondary tumours in her lungs. The acute emergency was managed but it was clear we had lost control and she would soon die. I felt sad for her and so inept, as I was not able to easily discuss with her what would happen to her and how she felt about it. Her parents came from their home overseas to be with her as she died and they sat with her husband by her hospital bed. I felt I could only observe their grief and was of little help. One afternoon Alice said to me 'I hope you do not feel you have let me down'. Whilst she was dying she was thinking about and trying to help me. She accepted I had done my best, inadequate as it may have been in my eyes. I think now that she had trusted me to do as well as I could for her, and valued this, and did not believe I had let her down.

One afternoon Alice said to me 'I hope you do not feel you have let me down'. Whilst she was dying she was thinking about and trying to help me.

What did Alice mean by 'let me down'? I believed I should have been able to talk more deeply with her and perhaps she was disappointed that I had not. To be let down suggests that another has not done enough, but at the same time has not left the sufferer feeling they have been personally diminished. The trust Alice placed in me was not imprudent but suggested to me her trust was not as broadly based and her expectations were less than if I had been her husband, a close friend or a parent. She expected care and understanding in a professional sense, and perhaps got more than this, but she did not see me in the same way as she would have a close friend. Nevertheless, I still could have betrayed her in a personal and professional sense if I had been indifferent or not acted to my full professional capacity.

Alice's trust included understanding and empathy for me, to which I responded. She maintained her personal control in our relationship, no matter how unequal it was in other ways and she had the freedom to care about me. She acknowledged my limitations and accepted I had done my best. She did something much greater than give forgiveness, she assured me I stood as an important person in her life and mattered for myself. Did I feel that I had let her down? No, I felt that we had all lost the battle together. Mostly I had realised that I had no real power as I could not control the disease, no matter what other powers Alice may have ceded to me. I had limited personal and professional skills and knowledge and knew I would always be vulnerable to ignorance and error. Yet I did not have the ability to talk through what she was feeling as she lay dying and it was not easy for me to acknowledge this and I did think I could have done better, and it made me aware of fate and happenstance and the fragility of all we try to do. I also eventually learnt that an inability to express something in mere words can be overcome in other ways. Because she had trusted me and understood why I had failed, Alice's dying gift to me was to say there was nothing for her to forgive and to release me of the responsibility I felt for her. The rewards for me were to know I had been appreciated and trusted and understood the value of that.

ALICE

You have cancer.
Harsh unhappy words,
insensitive, cruel.

Yet not as brutal as truth.
No euphemism will change the reality.
She accepts it calmly,
No tears, or none that I saw.

Deep in her eyes perhaps a dark shadow came.

She is young
with unusual vivacity.
Vibrant, warm
controlled
self assured.

She watches and jokes uncomfortably
as we plan the operation. Lines
drawn across soft, white, vulnerable flesh.
Does she feel our detachment then?

She let me do it. Always sickening
as the saw drags through the bone.
Primitive fear
overcome by a greater dread.
No detachment now.

Hide, hide the severed limb.
Yet later insist on its thorough dissection.

With the leg off we look forward.
Plan and fit the artificial limb.
Heavy, ungainly, inert.
Functional.

Now a team of helpers. So easy to
support and encourage, although we never
assuage the loss.

Strength she has,
greater courage than our heroes:
she reaches beyond fear.

Her innate joy gradually steals through
the outer gloom and overthrows it.

Months pass. We laugh.
Days of complacency near to happiness.
Absent fear is sufficient joy.
Relaxed.
The sharp bell crashes me awake,
An urgent voice.
I toss in bed whilst she breathes for life.
My sleep disturbed, hers destroyed.
That terrible disease has claimed her lungs.

I fail to meet her eyes.
She questions, asks for reasons.
None from me.

She dies. Yet too slowly.
Mother strong and vocal, artificial cheer.
Father numbly silent
painfully near.
Her husband
brooding, gaunt.
The men are fearfully still.

We are inept, faltering, helpless.
She, undaunted by the challenge of death
accepts pain and anguish with
cheerful strength.

The prosthesis lies by her bed unused.
The unwanted symbol of hope.
She hopes I do not feel I have let her down.

I try to reach her
yet cannot say the word.
She knows it
and lets me be.

The dominant models of medical ethics and the doctor–patient relationship look for some sort of covenant between rational people and overlook the importance of the emotional aspects of the relationship and the personal values and feelings of both the doctor and the patient. The idea of a covenant[2] emphasises principles such as promise keeping, autonomy and honesty, in the name of equality and individual rights, but it does not require of me that I should want to do things for others for their own sakes. Whilst I acknowledge the importance of rational equal relationships, we all still need to ask ourselves what sort of people we want to look after us when we are ill, frail or incompetent. Some years ago I heard a discussion on the radio in which it was acknowledged that the press usually presented the activities of doctors in one of two ways. Either the doctors were doing extraordinarily heroic and good things to help mankind, such as major joint replacements or cardiac transplants, or they were presented as very bad people who were 'ripping off the system', experimenting on patients without their knowledge or doing unnecessary surgery and other heinous things. It was suggested on the radio programme that these attitudes probably appeared because patients want to be able to trust their doctors. This trust is much easier if doctors are considered angels and the public has a perception of doctors being trustworthy and caring. On the other hand, if people do have this positive attitude to a doctor they will be very disappointed if they are let down and any misdemeanour or fault on the part of doctors may be considered a major breach of trust.

Debra Lupton[3] examined the recent movement to treat medical services as just another product to be consumed and doctors as simply suppliers of services. Lupton notes the emphasis on achieving patient satisfaction, but she questions whether this satisfaction may only mean some form of rational evaluation, judged dispassionately. Dispassionate judgement is based on an ideal of an individual being able to somehow distance himself from, and objectively assess, his own emotions and fears. Lupton points out recent sociological studies that claim the importance 'of acknowledging the complexity of the medical encounter on the interpersonal level and the tensions, ambivalences and contradictions that both patients and doctors may experience'. In her survey Lupton found a wide variation between how patients saw doctors, from severe criticism of them being money hungry and incompetent, to those who regarded doctors very well. However, there was a widespread emphasis on the individual's awareness of how they interacted with a doctor and if they felt the doctor had not treated them in a caring way, how the doctor appeared insensitive to their feelings or did not give them sufficient time to listen to their problems. 'Such doctors, it was contended, could not be trusted with one's health.'

The doctor–patient relationship does appear to be moving more towards one in which each individual respects the other's participation and humanity.

It is clear from Lupton's studies that most patients do not wish to have a close friendly relationship with their doctor and for some the maintenance of a 'professional distance' was seen as important. Nevertheless, this professional distance needed to be married to some empathy and concern for the patient. On the whole, patients placed much emphasis on the affective aspects of health care and saw emotional support and personal interest as important. The more articulate, better educated and younger patients were more inclined to wish for an equal relationship, in the sense that they became part of a team in which the patient seeks the help and expertise of the doctor. The doctor–patient relationship does appear to be moving more towards one in which each individual respects the other's participation and humanity, but Lupton insists it must also be seen that there are often emotional features to the relationship and dependency can be a central feature of illness as:

> Illness, disease, pain, disability and impending death, are
> all highly emotional states, and they all tend to encourage
> a need on the part of the suffering person for dependency
> upon another.

Whilst dependency on others may at times be seen as some form of weakness, being able to depend on others can at times be a great strength and comfort. While satisfaction with doctors generally means that patients trust that doctors acknowledge and accept a patient's autonomy and rights, it sometimes might 'spring from indulging a desire for dependence upon a paternalistic doctor, even as this confounds expectations around consumerism'.[4]

Whilst one of the aspects of a trusting relationship is that it makes the truster vulnerable, the contemporary American philosopher Martha Nussbaum[5] claims that the peculiar beauty of human excellence is its vulnerability. The good person is like a young plant, which, whilst it needs to be of good stock to grow well, is slender, fragile and in constant need of food from without. Like plants, humans need to live in a world that fosters their development. We could live without the help of friends; however love and friendship matter to us for their own sake and we cannot flourish without them. Yet one of the attributes we have as humans is to be able to reason and the application of this reason helps save us from living merely by luck. Nussbaum asks how can we be reliably good 'yet still be beautifully human?', in the sense that a purely rational being is likely to act carefully and prudently and not take risks, whilst acknowledging that by taking risks we can achieve much that is valuable in human existence. Nussbaum believes in the importance of rational decision-making, yet she recognises that:

> I must constantly choose among competing and apparently incommensurable goods and that circumstances may force me to a position where I cannot help being false to something or doing some wrong; that an event that simply happens to me may, without my consent, alter my life; that it is equally problematic to entrust one's good to friends, lovers or country and to try and have a good life without them – all these I take to be not just the material of tragedy, but everyday facts of lived practical reason.

But we sometimes trust too easily and without enough knowledge and thought. We are inclined to trust people such as used car salesmen, for example, and go along with their deals, even though experience tells us that we are likely to be badly used. Most of us are disposed to feel secure about the motives of public officials, institutions and individuals in a way that 'survives receiving a great deal of information about the incompetence, mendacity, greed, and so forth of some of them'.[6] If we respond to a betrayal of unthinking trust with outrage, this suggests it is important to us in spite of its apparent irrationality. It would seem certain, though, that there are some people we should rationally regard with a healthy suspicion. Whilst it is possible, at least for a while, to continue trusting somebody who has continually let us down, trusting in this way may shield and restrict us from fully appreciating a range of negative motives and emotions that others may have towards us, sometimes to our peril.

One of the core values of my profession is a commitment to teach our students and trainees. The first tenet of the Hippocratic Oath addresses this:

> I will pay the same respect to my master in the Science as to my parents and share my life with him and pay all my debts to him. I will regard his sons as my brothers and teach them the Science, if they desire to learn it, without fee or contract.

As a student and trainee surgeon I benefited from my seniors willingly and freely giving their time to teach me. I respected and admired my teachers and conscientiously carried on the tradition myself. I was proud of this tradition and boasted of our commitment to it.

In March 2015 a Sydney surgeon, Dr Gabrielle McMullin[7], publicly stated that a female trainee surgeon's career had been ruined after she won a sexual harassment case against a more senior male surgeon. Dr McMullin said junior female trainees would be better to give in to their male colleagues' sexual advances rather than complaining about them and 'realistically' would be better off giving them a 'blow job'. The junior surgeon, Dr Caroline Tan, stated that bullying, harassment and sexism is rife amongst surgeons and that the College of Surgeons should set up an independent body to hear complaints about misconduct and demonstrate that complainants would be listened to and protected.

My initial reaction to this news was that I had seen bullying and heard of sexual harassment by surgeons but thought they were uncommon. As a very junior trainee I was assisting a senior surgeon who was struggling with a difficult operation and who turned to me and said 'for this operation I need two experienced assistants and all I have is one bloody idiot'. I took it calmly and nothing further was said as I reasoned this was his reaction to stress and there was some truth in his statement, although I realise that if we had been equals he would not have got away with it so lightly. It was also, in my experience, a rare event. After the recent publicity about sexual harassment I asked two of my senior male colleagues if they had seen it and they both said no. My opinion was strengthened when the president of my surgical college stated he had not noticed it either. Fairly confident of my ground I broached the subject at a dinner party expecting a mild reaction. I was strongly criticised by two mature women, one of whom I soon discovered had been a sexual harassment officer at a university, whose understanding was quite different to mine. I was made to understand that such behaviour was not uncommon and could be very damaging to the victim. If this was the case, why had I not recognised it? And indeed, had I been a perpetrator?

There was worse to come.

Leaked documents[8] reveal Gabrielle McMullin told the college in 2008 that three female trainees had asked her advice on how to deal with senior surgeons asking for sexual favours. In two cases, corruption of training processes was alleged. 'In one case the surgeon has offered a place on a training scheme based on the granting of sexual services. In another case the surgeon has become very angry about the refusal of sexual services and consequently produced a report that questioned the ability of the trainee', Dr McMullin wrote to the then president. 'I have discussed, with my male colleagues, the possibility of making a complaint to the College and this suggestion has been greeted with horror and an assurance that such a complaint would mean the end of the surgical career of the trainee.' In the letter, Dr McMullin said she found the situation abhorrent and wanted to protect the trainees. She asked for advice about how the problem should be tackled. While her letter was acknowledged with a written response about the College's policies and a phone call, she said no one asked her who the alleged perpetrators were or for more information from the trainees. 'They did not want to know', she said. 'I was just a bad smell and they just wanted me to go away.' Documents show that in 2008, the College's chief executive, David Hillis, wrote to the executive committee describing Dr McMullin's claims as 'deeply disturbing', and he said college fellows had been involved in 'a number of events where professional (including educational) and personal activities have become significantly blurred'. Dr Hillis sought legal advice but it is unclear what, if anything, the College did in response to this.

My reaction to my senior colleague's emotional outburst in calling me a 'bloody idiot' was based on my belief that, no matter what he had said, whilst I was junior and inexperienced, I belonged as a member of his team. The next year he sent me a hand-written thank you note for attending his final hospital visit on his retirement and he gave me an excellent reference. I now know many of my female and Asian friends feel quite differently as they believe they do not fully belong in the team and feel they are seen as inferior and are treated differently. The problem is that whilst I now concede this, I was late to come to it and still do not really know what it is to walk in their shoes.

A former Victorian Police Commissioner, Ken Lay, commented on his experience of sexual harassment and bullying in the force.[9]

> Before standing down recently as Victoria's chief commissioner, I had seen worrying examples in Victoria Police where some men had used their position, and their sense of entitlement, to target women. These women were often junior in rank, and the advances were often characterised with a sexual intent, or the intent to demean or belittle. The Victoria Police executive simply had no means of determining the extent of the issues and the

damage it may be doing to some of our people. Yes, we had 'robust policies' and very clear guidelines, but often there was this underlying theme that would sometimes filter through to the highest levels of the organisation – sexual harassment was undereported, and victims were not prepared to report these matters because it could damage their career and damage them personally.

At times it is very difficult and painful for a proud organisation to accept criticism, particularly when it comes from within. Instinctively it is sometimes easier to deny, to attack the messenger, or to roll out myriad 'best practice' policies to defend one's good name. Sometimes, however, looking in the mirror and reflecting on the ugliness that may be present will make organisations better, people safer, and build community confidence.

Gabrielle McMullin was criticised by many women for her remarks, but she knew exactly how to move her male colleagues and get them to act quickly. The College vowed to work to solve the problem and put in place an interim process to manage complaints about discrimination, bullying and sexual harassment. They set up an independent 'expert group' to study and advise on the problem. Pending further advice from the expert group they ensured fellows, trainees and international medical graduates had access to a program to support people who have been subject to discrimination, bullying or sexual harassment. As a priority, the expert group promoted opportunities for interested stakeholders to engage with its work and share their experiences. In September 2015 the groups' report found sexual harassment and sexism were major problems for the College and there was a lack of trust in complaints' handling and a demonstrable lack of consequences for perpetrators.

As I learnt from Alice, trust works in more than one way. In a good relationship we learn from each other, perhaps more so if we are verbally articulate and emotionally aware of each other. This is not easy in an unequal relationship, more so if we are blind to another's needs and selfishly put ourselves first. It is useful to be able look into a mirror, but we only see our image of ourselves. It is more important to see ourselves through the eyes of others. As surgeons we have not yet looked deeply into Ken Lay's mirror, or more crucially, into the eyes of our juniors, and our patients, to see there how we should behave to enable them to trust us.

It is useful to be able look into a mirror, but we only see our image of ourselves. It is more important to see ourselves through the eyes of others.

Nussbaum[10] has commented on problems young men have in the USA:

> A large proportion of boys are quite unable to talk about how they feel and how others feel – because they have learned to be ashamed of feelings and needs, and to push them underground. But that means that they don't know how to deal with their own emotions, or to communicate them to others. When they are frightened, they don't know how to say it, or even to become fully aware of it. Often they turn their own fear into aggression.

Carol-Anne Moulton,[11] a Fellow of my College, believes that there is a surgical stereotype: that of machismo, certainty, bravery and confidence, and that many surgeons try to live up to it but 'fall short of this in their inner sense of self'. Moulton believes the stereotype does not truly exist in most surgeons and is simply a front that 'we try to live up to, or pretend to embody'. She believes there are benefits in the surgical stereotype, as a belief in oneself can lead to effort, perseverance and success – and seeing ourselves mirrored in this image, surrounded by a team that believes in us, reinforces the stereotype. Moulton calls this a 'looking-glass self', an idea we will see has its roots extending back through the German philosopher Hegel to Plato. She believes the stereotype can be useful as the front exudes a confidence when dealing with patients that engenders trust. However, a false front can be most untrustworthy. Moulton does not believe that the increasing number of female surgeons has changed things much yet, as they have tended to take on the dominant male culture. She feels that the feminine traits, also felt by men, are mostly hidden and need to be displayed and 'for this to happen the profession would have to change its value system', which 'may also require changes in public expectations of surgeons as I believe this is also a driver behind the stereotype'. Moulton suspects that:

> Most surgeons would be more competent, safer and happier if we were to begin to understand these social-cultural influences on our decision making. I think we'd be happier when we begin to see that 'faking' something we do not feel can eat away at us and prevent us from seeking help when we need to, such as debriefing after a complication, for example. If we understand the pressures on us, we are then in a better position to make deliberate choices of how to act professionally and respond emotionally.

We are constantly trying to improve and have an extensive ongoing education program. There are courses on communication, people skills, motivational needs, recognising stress in oneself and colleagues, non-technical skills, teaching skills and managing trainees, as well as the mainstream technical skills and continuing education. There is a booklet on bullying and harassment. None of these work if we do not truly see the problem. The booklet on bullying is freely available but we do not think it applies to us. Just as importantly, however, have I mistreated and betrayed my patients and not recognised it?

I am a member of a professional body presently feeling the heat of public disapprobation because we do not fully see a problem ...

Alice was one of a number of important people in my personal and professional life who taught me to see and hear others more clearly and who helped me develop some empathy and understanding of another's suffering. In doing this I have learnt a lot about myself. I have a lot yet to learn. I am a member of a professional body presently feeling the heat of public disapprobation because we do not fully see a problem and those aspects which we did see we brushed aside until attention was forced upon us. I know we are not alone. All organisations are probably like us.

Throughout this book I try to simply and clearly explain how certain philosophers and their ideas can guide us to understand how best we can live and practise. One of these is Socrates, who suggested that we do not need to despair:

Plato:[12] *Phaedo, 89d–90a. The Last days of Socrates*

'Misanthropy creeps in as a result of placing too much trust in someone without having the knowledge required: we suppose the person to be completely genuine, sound and trustworthy, only to find a bit later that he's bad and untrustworthy, and then it happens again with someone else; when we've experienced the same thing many times over, and especially when it's with those we'd have supposed our nearest and dearest, we get fed up with making so many mistakes and so end up hating everyone and supposing no one to be sound in any respect. Haven't you seen this happening?'

'Yes, certainly,' I said.

'Not a pretty thing, then,' said Socrates 'and clearly someone like that will have been trying to handle human relationships without the knowledge he needs, of what humans are like; for I imagine if he had been doing it on the basis of a proper understanding, he would have supposed things to be as they really are, with the very good and the very bad forming a small minority, and the majority in the middle between good and bad.'

We can all be angels or villains. How can Socrates' understanding that we are usually neither help us to manage the villains and get closer to the angels?

When I trained as a surgeon I developed a way of thinking that appeared to serve me well in that trade. I found that studying ethics and philosophy required me to learn to think quite differently. It took quite a while to learn what amounted to a new language and even longer to expand the way I saw the world. Whilst surgery often appears to be practical and pragmatic, it is also complex and uncertain, and we usually make decisions based on our idea of probability rather than true knowledge. Yet we are asked to give clear advice and guidance and act with calm certainty. We appear to be what we are not and, not surprisingly, we then come to act as we appear to be, rather than what we are.

When I trained as a surgeon I developed a way of thinking that appeared to serve me well in that trade. I found that studying ethics and philosophy required me to learn to think quite differently.

In this book I build an argument for the importance and the nature of the trustworthy doctor. In doing this I analyse the meaning of trust in its rational, emotional, social and biological aspects. I explain how an understanding of the strong emotions associated with an awareness of betrayal emphasises the fundamental importance of trust to us. I use my own experiences in clinical practice to explore the nature of trustworthiness in healthcare, but this could also guide others in other aspects of life. There are many forms of betrayal in medical practice, some apparently trivial, but important nevertheless. There are also differences between betraying someone and simply making a mistake, but sometimes how we react to and manage mistakes can turn them into betrayals. After a betrayal comes the possibility of forgiveness, mostly of others, sometimes of ourselves. Forgiveness can be healing if it is thoughtful and whole-hearted, but risky nevertheless, and needs to be covered by the arch of justice.

There are also differences between betraying someone and simply making a mistake, but sometimes how we react to and manage mistakes can turn them into betrayals.

This book owes much to philosophy, but it also includes something of the trials and triumphs of medicine and a splattering of science. It required honesty and courage because sometimes I lay myself and my colleagues bare. It is the experiences of many patients, friends and colleagues that inspires the narrative behind the humanity in this book. Many of the stories developed from events in my own life or those I have shared with others. Tales that involve patients, whose privacy is sacrosanct, whilst based on real events, have been changed so that no one person can be recognised.

Chapter Two: Trust and the Possibility of Betrayal

I remember travelling on a suburban train in Melbourne, Australia, when I was ten years old. The carriage was old and not air-conditioned and the windows were open to let in fresh air. There was a girl of about my age sitting in the seat opposite me and as we neared my destination she bent forward and asked me to show her my ticket. Without thinking I gave it to her and she promptly threw it out the window. I was aghast, as in those days there was always an official at the station waiting to collect the tickets. I feared my own shame and the disappointment my parents would feel if I was caught, apparently travelling without a ticket. Fortunately, I was able to hide behind a shed at the station until the ticket-collector went back into his office and thus made my escape. It appeared to me at the time that no harm was done, yet I still feel the guilt almost as sharply now as I felt it then, even though I was innocent. Even more, I remember the simple trust I had in that girl and my dismay when she betrayed it.

Twenty-five years later I was a junior consultant surgeon at a large teaching hospital in Melbourne. I had been on call the previous night and all the members of the orthopaedic unit were reviewing the patients who had been admitted and treated under my care. One of our surgical registrars had telephoned me during the previous night for advice on the management of a patient and I had agreed to his suggested treatment. It was clear on reviewing our decision the following morning that another course of action would have been preferable. The registrar was questioned about his actions and he turned towards me and said that I had agreed to it. I denied this and said he must have been mistaken. I lied and put my reputation before his. My memory of his reaction is burnt into my soul and I can still see the hurt in his eyes. I had betrayed him and I am sure he never trusted me again. Probably, he was wary of trusting other consultants in the future. My guilt lives with me still, even though I made sure I never did such a thing again, no matter at what cost to my personal and professional image.

For many years I was an orthopaedic surgeon and I often discussed surgical procedures and their associated risks with my patients. My decision to explore the meaning and value of trust began some twenty-five years ago when I was explaining to a patient the various complications of a certain operation. She interrupted me to say, 'I don't need to know all that, I trust you.' I thought it remarkable that she should say this as we had met for the first time only twenty minutes previously. If hers had been an isolated case then I may have thought less about it, as it was not exceptional for a patient to say something like that. Acknowledging the importance most of us give to having some say in and control over what happens to us, particularly if it might harm us, I began to reflect on what it was that motivated her to surrender some of this control to me. What did she mean when she said she trusted me and what brought her to do so? Was there anything about me as a person she trusted or did I, perhaps, simply represent a professional whom she thought it was safe to trust because of my position?

My initial reaction had been to feel somewhat flattered that I was considered somebody of such good character as to be trustworthy, but this emotional response was soon followed by a realisation that she had placed some burden upon me. For some reason I felt strongly that I had to be worthy of her trust. If my patient was to abrogate her right to be as fully informed as possible, how did that affect my obligation to her? In some ways it seemed that by offering her trust to me she reduced my responsibilities, as I did not have to give her all the information she may have needed to make a properly informed decision. But she had also placed an added responsibility upon me that was separate from, and in addition to, my normal duty to make sure she had enough information to give fully informed consent for her operation. She was taking a risk in trusting me as I could omit significant factors that may have been in her best interests to know. I now believed I was expected to take on the responsibility of acting well towards somebody who trusted me, simply because of that trust. In my superficial assessment of her trust I felt at least two things. Firstly, a moral obligation to her and secondly, an emotional response to the trust she had placed in me. It made me feel good and want to be good. It did not occur to me then that I might also betray her trust.

In life we often make decisions and take risks. If we enter a relationship with a surgeon these risks can be quite significant and sometimes life threatening. It is plainly prudent to minimise risks and, as much as possible, to insist on some form of accountability from those we deal with. As human relationships are often unequal, protecting the weaker party from the stronger may require some sort of social artifice and one way of doing this is to have a formal contract that is protected by the law and by legal redress if things go awry. I wondered if it might not be better if my patient and I entered into some form of a contract protecting both of us through a regulated agreement that fully acknowledged her rights, my duties and our joint responsibilities. There are, of course, other ways of regulating unequal relationships outside of a strictly legal regime. These include general conventions to behave in particular ways, social obligations, moral principles, duties espoused by organisations and the feeling of individual responsibility that one person may have for another. Another way is through a trusting relationship, which perhaps could include all of these things. That my patient chose a path involving trust suggests she believed there were some benefits in trusting that made it worthwhile to take a risk with me. What were those benefits and what was the risk?

However capable or powerful a person is, when she takes the role of a patient she becomes the weaker partner. I use the term 'patient', which is derived from a Latin word meaning 'to suffer', as I believe it is an appropriate term and it is not demeaning. Some use the term 'client', but this comes from another Latin root that means to obey or to be subordinate, and in Roman usage this meant a plebeian under the control of a patrician, the very opposite to valuing a person's autonomy. Using the word 'patient' emphasises that in the relationship the doctor is dealing with somebody who is suffering and who may need special consideration and compassion. I use the term 'doctor' to include all qualified medical practitioners. The healing professions include many others: nurses, physiotherapists, social workers, technicians and paramedics, to name just a few. I see them as part of my world and they too are embraced in this book as equal health professionals.

Hegel,[13] the eighteenth-century German philosopher, described personal trust in this way:

> I can trust a person if I believe he has sufficient insight to treat my cause as if it were his own and to deal with it in the light of his own best knowledge and conscience.

Hegel's definition of trust is a personal one and he sees trust as an integral part of a relationship between two people. The person I trust is expected to try and put himself in my position and assume my values and aspirations and act upon these as well as he can, as he thinks I would wish him to act. I mostly tend to think of trust as part of a relationship between two individuals, but we often include small groups as constituting a trusting relationship providing there are significant personal relationships within the group. This could be between members of a team or a small group of people with a common goal. Trust in a personal sense can be contrasted with a general non-personal trust I might have to a profession, such as a group of accountants or doctors, or an institution like a hospital. If I am to include large organisations in my attempt to understand trust, I will need to expand Hegel's definition to decide whether a large institution can be considered as trustworthy or whether I should be content with thinking of institutions only in terms of reliability. Thus I need to distinguish between trust and reliability.

When someone decides to trust another person it seems likely that they believe they are dealing with a person worthy of their trust. There is a dimension of respected judgement and character in the person whom we describe as 'trustworthy' that is not present when we describe someone as merely 'reliable'. We admire people of good character and good will and these are presumably some of the features of a trustworthy person. In contradistinction, the vision we have of people we label 'untrustworthy', as opposed to 'unreliable', suggests the connotations of those two words are strikingly different. This may be particularly so in unequal relationships, like the medical one, where the patient's outcome may depend on the personal attributes of the doctor.

When we trust and are let down we do not feel disappointment, as we might if a machine let us down; we feel betrayed.

When we trust and are let down we do not feel disappointment, as we might if a machine let us down; we feel betrayed. We take a particular kind of attitude towards someone we trust, called a 'reactive attitude'. [14, 15] A reactive attitude is an attitude we take in response to our interpretation of another's attitude to us. These are those attitudes that we normally take towards people, rather than towards machines, changes in the weather or other natural phenomena. Attitudes such as resentment, when someone lets us down, or gratefulness, when they help, are examples of attitudes that we feel towards people when they act in certain ways, particularly when we believe they have some moral responsibility for what they do. In betrayal the attitude is not only towards the other's lack of goodwill but also to their regard. We have a readiness to feel betrayed if our trust is disappointed and it is this stance that makes the difference between reliance and trust. Trusting somebody does not involve merely having a belief about them, but also includes expecting them to do something and being prepared to feel betrayed if they do not. Trusting someone involves treating them as a person and one does not take a participant stance towards a non-person. Thus at least some forms of trust are part of personal relationships, with accompanying affective attitudes in which the truster at least may feel that emotion plays a significant part.

The trustee may also take a particular type of attitude towards the truster.[16] Trust is an attitude of optimism, concerned amongst other things with the goodwill of the one being trusted and the idea that the trustee will be 'favourably moved' by the thought that we are counting on them. The optimism is not one of looking on the bright side of life in general, but of having some confidence that the person they are trusting has some goodwill towards them. This confidence is an affective attitude, rather than a judgement of the facts they know or believe about the trustee as a trustworthy person. The trusted person will be favourably moved by the thought that someone is in some way including them in a personal relationship. The truster is thus expecting the trustee to form some kind of affective attitude towards them. Any affectivity the trustee may feel could also include the enjoyment of the goodwill of the truster, particularly if they value the good opinion of the truster, and this may actually increase their trustworthiness as they desire to please.[17] The opposite also applies. If the trustee does not care about the opinion of the truster then the truster may be less trustworthy unless they have another reason to be trustworthy –for instance, identification with an institution that depends on trust, or a wish to have a good opinion of themselves as a trustworthy person. At times the trustee may find the expectations of a truster unwelcome and whilst we would probably never object to someone thinking of us as a trustworthy person, we may object to others trusting us when we would rather they did not.

Some patients too willingly hand over their responsibility and are too quick to blame others if they do not achieve their desired outcome. Good trusting relations involve both parties and should include some responsibility for thought and action, even from the less powerful party. I was once on a panel selecting young doctors to train as orthopaedic surgeons. The candidates were asked how they would respond to a patient who asked not to be fully informed; rather like my patient. The candidates' answer was invariably that they would not completely accept the patient's attitude and would insist on them knowing at least the most common and more dangerous complications of a procedure. The candidates reasoned that a patient has some responsibility for their own fate and ought not to delegate this entirely to another.

Trust in personal relationships usually involves making choices about the giving of something valuable to another. This may be anything that we possess, hold dear or care for and which has significant meaning to us. It includes information that is relevant to our wellbeing, promise keeping and veracity. The trusting person, the truster, relies on the goodwill of the person who is being trusted, the trustee, and thus becomes vulnerable to the consequent power of the trustee. As we have seen, a trusting relationship has an added dimension, in that the truster also takes, or is disposed to take, a certain attitude to the trustee and perhaps also the trustee may take a certain attitude to the truster. This attitude may include an emotional response and an expectation of how each person ought to behave. The personal trust I have in mind refers to that which occurs when a person says or implies 'I will trust you.' The truster should have sincerely considered the meaning of this statement and has asked themselves the question 'Ought I trust you?'[18] This further implies that they have some choice in the matter, that they have thought about it and that they are thinking rationally. The statement 'I will trust you' should mean that I have considered the situation in which I have something valuable that I cannot or choose not to look after myself, and I have decided to give it to you to look after. I make a free choice to give it to you. My choice includes my assessment of its value to me and your worthiness and ability to look after it.

Excluded from this version of personal trust are statements like 'You give me no choice but to trust you'. The fact that I say, 'I am given no choice' means that my options are limited or I believe that I am being coerced into trusting you, as this is not an action of my own free will but one that has been forced upon me by some external power or set of circumstances. It might even be unreasonable to use the word 'rely' in this situation, as to say 'you give me no choice but to rely on you' also suggests an action that is beyond my control. It might be a better statement to say 'I am in your power and am unable to influence what you do but I hope that you will look after my valuables as I would like' or 'I am forced to depend on you'. Obviously, trust is rarely thought about in this way. We often trust people without apparently thinking about it much or at all.

When people trust doctors they are likely to expect more of them than they do of police officers or airline pilots. This is not to diminish the critical importance that the police and others whom we depend on should be trustworthy, but because of the degree of intimacy in the doctor–patient relationship, where secrets, vices and weaknesses can be exposed.

These are also exposed to the police, lawyers and many other professionals but are seen in different ways. Patients are at a disadvantage because of their ill health and may feel powerless and uncertain, and need to be able to trust the doctor in a way they do not trust policemen or pilots. This makes the relationship particularly vulnerable to any suspicion or suggestion of betrayal and it makes it very easy for patients to come to distrust doctors if things go wrong.

When people trust doctors they are likely to expect more of them than they do of police officers or airline pilots.

In personal trusting relationships the truster voluntarily gives some power to the trustee over his goods. The voluntary nature of this type of trust can be implied, as I can place myself in a situation where I can expect the person with whom I am relating to behave as though we are in a trusting relationship. Examples of this would include that between a priest and a parishioner or a doctor and a patient, unless it is agreed otherwise. A patient does not necessarily have to tell their doctor that they trust them, as trust is usually assumed in this relationship, and the doctor is expected to act as well as they can in their patient's best interest. Most would say absolute and blind trust however, was imprudent, as to act well in a patient's best interest a doctor needs to know what the patient's real and full interests are and the patient may also want to know something about the doctor to see if they are worthy of their trust.

The danger for those who decide to trust another is that they may be betrayed. Most of us know this and we tend to choose those whom we trust carefully, and thus we may need to share the responsibility if we are let down, as we have freely chosen to trust someone when we might have chosen otherwise. This responsibility may include a patient who, whilst choosing to trust, does not sufficiently explore their own preferences, or a young boy who hands over a ticket to a stranger without thinking through what could happen next. Hard experience is often the only way we can know this and reflection may give us the wisdom to manage better in the future. There are times when we are especially vulnerable and feel that we are owed trust because of this. Betrayal in these circumstances can be devastating.

The type of trust I have discussed so far describes us making conscious, discriminating choices. Recently I was hurrying along a street near my home, hoping not to miss my train, when a man accosted me and asked me for the time. Without thinking, I stopped, looked at my watch and told him, correctly, that it was 9.47. It did not occur to me to react in any other way and he accepted my information without question. If I had told the stranger the incorrect time and he subsequently missed an appointment, would this be an example of betrayal? As I had no particular relationship with this person, then, at first sight at least, I don't think that I would say that I had betrayed him, even though I can imagine he would be resentful and perhaps angry. Yet, an emotional response like this surely indicates that the interaction must, in my mind at least, have meant something to the stranger, so maybe there is often some unconscious trust present between strangers and therefore the potential for betrayal. Was there some 'implicit' trust between me and the girl on the train? I certainly felt strongly that I had in some way been wounded by her and, although I have never before considered she had betrayed me, perhaps in some social sense she did. I think it unlikely she considered she had betrayed me and I can only guess at her motivation; maybe it was a tease to get a reaction or perhaps a show of power. If it was to do with power it may be a good example of how power can be thoughtlessly used to harm others, perhaps without the powerful being aware of the potential for betrayal and its long-lasting effects. In my betrayal of my registrar I was certainly aware of my power. My motives were purely selfish, as I did not want to seem inexperienced or foolish in front of my senior colleagues and did not yet have the courage to expose myself. I have since learnt that the harm I caused, to myself as well as my registrar, far outweighed any benefit for me at the time. There is nothing intrinsically wrong in making mistakes or having poor judgment providing you reflect and learn from your experience. There is a great deal wrong in deliberately betraying someone, particularly if he is relatively powerless and vulnerable.

If the idea of betrayal comes from the loss or failure of trust, this implies some disappointment in the expectation of a benevolent action or failure by the trustee to acknowledge the importance of the truster. The idea of betrayal implies a prescriptive sense, in that we believe the betrayer ought not to be behaving or thinking in a particular way. Betrayal does not appear to be a purely descriptive concept, that is, purely describing what has happened without any judgment of it being right or wrong. Nor is it one of indifference. Indeed, if a friend were to seriously betray me I may think the betrayal was in itself sufficient to end the friendship.

Most of us have personal relationships in which we remain trustful despite the known untrustworthiness of others. These include an unfaithful spouse, a wayward child or an alcoholic lover, amongst others. For example, consider that you are the parent of an irresponsible child. Your son is a teenager and you are paying him an allowance, as he is a student, however he is spending his money on alcohol and drugs and is not attending to his studies. He is still living at home and his behaviour is erratic and destructive. He asks you for his regular allowance, claiming that he has 'turned the corner' and he will study and no longer take drugs or drink to excess. This has happened before and your friends and relatives tell you that you should not trust him, as he will only spend the money unwisely again. You argue that you give your son money, shelter and food simply because he is your son and you love him and need to protect him as he needs help. It may also be true that you give him money because you *want* to trust him and have not yet given up hope that he will learn to be trustworthy. Even though you are disappointed in his behaviour you continually give him another chance. As a parent you value trust and go on offering your son the opportunity to be trustworthy long after outsiders have told you that your behaviour is irrational. He is also probably aware that he is behaving in an untrustworthy way and you understand that teenagers often feel guilty about this. Neither you nor your son wish to accept that he cannot be trusted and you go on trusting him when it no longer appears rational to do so. As a parent you admit it is irrational but stress the value of trust and how important it is to you. As a parent you show a commitment to your relationship with your son and also want to show him you value him as a person. You are also inclined to trust in his intentions to behave better, even though you know he is not able to put his intentions to good practice and therefore you show him you value his goodness no matter how fragile this is. Often parental trust of this type is vindicated as the child grows older. If it is, then your son may feel better about himself as he realises your love and the value you have continually placed upon him as a person. Thus sometimes we trust in a rather non-rational way, which feels like real trust to us and of value in itself. Yet often we have seen a child take advantage of a parent's love and sacrifice, and continue to live selfishly.

Sometimes we give trust as a gift of love, as we do for our wayward son. We are not acting rationally if we are thinking only of the outcome in the short term, but we may be if we believe that trusting relationships have value in themselves. We show the value of trust to our children by teaching them both to trust and be trustworthy. As a child grows and learns about his parents he may increasingly make conscious choices to trust them in particular circumstances. For a child learning about trust the failure of a particular trust may be very important even though giving away something like a small secret might appear trivial to an adult. Persistent failure in trusting relationships, no matter how trivial, may make the child suspicious of all relationships so that they grow up untrusting and unable to make good friendships. Thus the trustee has some moral responsibility in two ways. Firstly, to care sympathetically for the weaker party and secondly, to create a climate of trust in which personal relationships can flourish. If we are sensible parents, we do not expect too much of our children and realise that trusting relationships have to be learnt and developed gradually and within the capacity of the person. We also spend time teaching our children to be trustworthy by giving them tasks within their capabilities, praising them when they are successful and showing some displeasure when they are not.

As a surgeon I noticed that if I found myself in a situation where I believed I was not being trusted I felt inadequate and I was inclined to conclude that I was not performing well or not being as approachable or as sensitive as I ought to be. This could, of course, be the correct interpretation and suggests that I needed to improve my performance. Any loss of confidence I might have had led me to be less certain about my relationship with the patient, but also to be less certain about their condition and less certain about the advice I gave. Not being trusted tends to make me defensive. I was reluctant to offer advice in case it was taken the wrong way and worried if the outcome was unsatisfactory the patient would blame me. A patient who did not trust me was unlikely to forgive any error of judgement I might make, even if that error was made in good faith and was the best possible judgement that could have been made considering the circumstances. Usually if I sensed a patient did not trust me I persevered until I believed they did. Occasionally I had to suggest to a patient that our relationship was unlikely to be professionally or personally satisfactory and recommended that someone else treat them. The situation I could not resolve occurred when a patient did not trust me and I was not aware of it.

The practice of medicine is a good and important example of the place of trust in our lives but trust has a profound and pervasive presence throughout everything we do and value.

Trust has advantages and risks and imposes an obligation on the trustee, and perhaps the truster, and it may be associated with complex emotional responses. It is my view that trust is and should be central to the doctor–patient relationship. This is often generally accepted but rarely analysed and the concepts of trust and betrayal in medicine are not usually well taught or centrally presented in courses on medical ethics, nor given much credence in legal circles. I will examine the meaning and significance of trust and betrayal using examples from the experiences of both doctors and patients. The practice of medicine is a good and important example of the place of trust in our lives but trust has a profound and pervasive presence throughout everything we do and value and I will take some time to examine it in the wider context of everyday life. I will show that the tendency to ignore, downplay or bypass trust in medical practice must not be easily set aside. It has implications for legal, social and contractual approaches to medical ethics and practice because these approaches, while important, do not reflect the actual reality of medical practice. Trust, with its concomitant less rational but human dimensions such as human sympathy and caring, is a better starting point.

Chapter Three: Practical Wisdom and Human Frailty

When I was a junior surgical registrar a young man, Frank, was admitted to our orthopaedic unit. He had a malignant cartilage tumour growing from a bone in his pelvis. These tumours, known as chondrosarcomas, are unusual malignancies in that they grow very slowly and rarely metastasise, that is, spread to other areas of the body. They grow slowly because their tissue is poorly vascularised and there are relatively few active cells dispersed amongst the substance of cartilage. Chondrosarcomas cause damage through relentless growth in a local area. A tumour such as this in the pelvis will gradually increase in size until it compresses the blood vessels, nerves and other structures, such as the ureters carrying urine into the pelvis from the kidneys to the bladder. This compression eventually leads to severe pain, weakness, incontinence, infection, kidney failure and death. Currently the best way we know how to treat these tumours is to excise them with a relatively wide margin of normal tissue around them. As these tumours are slow growing and often quite large before they cause noticeable symptoms they may require surgery that is extremely destructive. Nowadays, with better technology and increasing skills we are able to excise at least half the pelvis and reconstruct the pelvic girdle and in doing so preserve the leg. When I was young the only way we could treat these tumours was to do a very radical operation, called a hind-quarter amputation, in which the whole leg, the hip joint and that half of the pelvic bones were removed. This was very major surgery and very few surgeons had the skills and experience to do it.

Frank had a large chondrosarcoma on one side of his pelvis. His only symptom was a vague feeling of discomfort in the region of his hip and lower abdomen and he had felt a firm mass in his buttock. The senior orthopaedic surgeon arranged with an experienced abdominal surgeon to do the operation together. The operation was performed one afternoon and took approximately three hours. I was not at the operation as I was assisting another surgeon in a different procedure in an adjoining operating theatre but I understood that the operation had gone well. After dinner I decided to go to the ward and see how Frank was, even though there was a more junior resident on call for the orthopaedic unit. I asked Frank how he felt and he said he was feeling well but he was having a lot of pain in his leg. I replied that this was not unusual and was known as phantom pain, a condition where a patient who has lost a limb can still feel the limb, which may be painful. 'Oh no Doc,' he said, 'It's my other leg, my good leg.'

Nearly fifty years later, whilst I cannot remember much else about him, I can still remember pulling back his bedclothes and examining his remaining limb. It was pale, cold, numb and pulseless. There was no blood getting to his remaining good leg and it was dying. I rang the operating surgeon who had just arrived home after completing his patient rounds. We agreed that the most likely diagnosis was a clot, or thrombosis, in the arteries in the pelvis that supplied the remaining good leg. He said he would come in immediately and asked me to contact a vascular surgeon and arrange an operating theatre straight away. By the time we were all assembled and the patient was anaesthetised in theatre, it was about nine o'clock at night. The vascular surgeon made a small incision into the main femoral artery of the remaining leg and passed a catheter up and down. He found no evidence of a clot but there was no blood flowing down the artery. He pushed the catheter further up the artery and suddenly met a firm obstruction. Whatever was blocking the artery it did not appear to be a clot. We prepared the abdomen to explore, by open surgery, the blood vessels in the pelvis. The fresh arterial blood that supplies the pelvis and the lower limbs comes down the aorta, which is the main artery leading from the heart and runs at the back of the abdominal cavity, nestled to the left of the spine. Not far below where it gives off the arteries to the kidneys, the aorta divides into two and each branch is called the common iliac artery. A few centimetres later the artery divides again into two, one branch being the internal iliac artery, which supplies the organs in the pelvis and the surrounding muscles and bone, and the other the external iliac artery that enters the leg and becomes the femoral artery, which supplies almost all the blood to the leg. In performing a hind-quarter amputation this area is approached from the upper thigh, groin, buttock and lower abdomen. The surgeons go from the superficial aspect deeper and deeper into the pelvis, exposing layer after layer of tissue, dividing and removing bone and soft tissues to eventually reach and identify the various iliac arteries. This is quite difficult to do, particularly if there is a large solid tumour compressing and distorting the tissues around it. You cannot see clearly what is deep to you until you are right upon it. The operation requires prolonged concentration and meticulous attention to detail.

The surgeons had planned to tie a ligature around the common iliac artery and then divide the vessels below this, thus removing most of the half of the pelvis and the tumour and the leg below it in one block. We started exploring the area by identifying the lower aorta and discovered that the surgeons had made a major error. They had tied off the lower aorta above where it divides into the iliac vessels, which meant they had also blocked the blood supply to the other side of the pelvis and the good limb. The vascular surgeon cut through the ligature at the lower end of the aorta and blood immediately began to fill the common iliac vessel below it. The time was 10 pm. The aorta had been ligatured at about 3 pm that afternoon so the whole limb had been without a blood supply for about seven hours. The vascular surgeon passed a catheter down the arterial system of the remaining leg and it appeared to pass easily, confirming that there was no other obstruction in the main vessels. After we had sewn up the abdomen and removed the drapes, we examined the leg. It was still cold and pale. A pulse could be felt over the femoral artery in the groin but none lower. We had no choice but to wait and see. I finished some chores, saw a number of patients and slept overnight in the residents' quarters. The next morning I was up early to see the patient. He told me that his leg was still painful and mostly numb but he could feel bits of it. I examined him and the leg was not totally numb or totally cold. There was blotchy discolouration throughout and, pressing the skin of his lower leg I could just make it blanch, suggesting there was some small blood flow. The pulses around the ankle and foot were absent. Over the next few days he gradually improved, the colour, sensation and function slowly returned, and after a week his leg appeared to have returned almost to normal. He went home on crutches with an appointment to see a prosthetist.

I learnt many things from that case, one of which is that in a fit young person you can shut off the blood supply to the leg for many hours and sometimes get away with it. I also learnt that even the most experienced and competent surgeons can and do make mistakes. Furthermore, this was a mistake they had not imagined they would make and almost certainly would not have warned the patient that it could happen. In 1966, when this happened, we did not recognise the concept of informed consent and it is very unlikely that Frank would have been told much about the surgery or the risks. He would have been aware of the diagnosis and some of the prognosis otherwise he would not have consented to have the surgery. Consent in those days did not include signing a form or contain any reference to any possible complications, as it was considered that if a patient turned up for an operation that was consent enough. Nevertheless, even now the possibility of an error of this type and severity probably would not be mentioned, because it is so rare, unless the patient specifically asked about it. Surgeons, like all humans, sometimes make major mistakes that they do not imagine could happen. If Frank had lost his good leg he would have been severely disabled and almost certainly confined to a wheel chair with all the psychological, physical and medical problems that entails. The surgeons would have felt very badly about it but I doubt if they would have considered they had betrayed him.

Surgeons, like all humans, sometimes make major mistakes that they do not imagine could happen.

In another place and much later time Robert left work early. It was his twenty-sixth birthday and as he steered his motorbike out onto the wet road he thought of Wendy, his pregnant wife, who would not yet be home from work, and he anticipated the smile in her eyes if he was there to greet her. It was a warm, wet, tropical night and she had booked a table at a restaurant overlooking the sea for a special dinner. His work as an electrician was going well and they could comfortably afford it. As he entered an intersection the sun was low in his eyes and he did not see the moving shape until it was too late. Applying his brakes hard, he skidded on the slippery road and the bike went from under him, crushing his leg as he slid and slammed into a moving, unyielding bus. In one way he was lucky, an ambulance was soon at the scene, he was efficiently assessed and splinted, dressings were applied, intravenous fluids commenced and he reached our hospital emergency department within a 'golden hour'. The so-called 'golden hour' refers to good evidence that if resuscitation is commenced and the patient brought to an emergency centre within an hour of a severe injury he is much more likely to survive than if it is delayed longer. In the emergency department Robert was pale, sweaty, had low blood pressure and a fast weak pulse; signs of severe blood loss. The most obvious external injury was a fracture of his lower left leg. The leg had been twisted and dragged along the ground, skin had been torn and ground off, and pieces of bone, muscle and tendon were clearly visible in the wound. The wound was severely contaminated with his clothing and gravel from the road surface. His foot was a greyish-blue colour and it was not possible to feel the arterial pulses around his ankle and foot. Insufficient blood was getting through to his foot to maintain viability and he was in danger of losing his leg and, if not quickly treated, his life.

Robert was conscious but drowsy. He moaned with pain but was able to state that, whilst his foot felt very numb, he could just feel it when it was touched. As resuscitation was continued with intravenous fluids and oxygen he was kept warm with thermal blankets and a primary assessment was made as to his general condition. He did not have any major head, neck or chest injury. He complained of tenderness in his abdomen, which appeared distended. He had many abrasions and he had a dislocated big toe in his right foot. The primary investigations confirmed the shattered left tibia and fibula bones and indicated the strong possibility of bleeding in the abdomen. In spite of continuing resuscitation and urgent blood transfusion, Robert's blood pressure remained low and his pulse rate only reduced slightly.

I was the orthopaedic surgeon on call that night. My registrar had been called to the emergency department soon after Robert had arrived and had already assessed his leg, organised appropriate X-rays and liaised with the emergency staff and the general surgical registrar. I arrived in the emergency department at the same time as the abdominal surgeon. We agreed that Robert needed exploratory surgery to the abdomen and that this should precede surgery for his leg, as he would have quickly bled to death if nothing were done. We told Robert briefly what we planned to do and asked him if he agreed to it. He was in pain, shocked and receiving strong pain-relieving medication and we did not expect him to fully understand what was about to happen.

In the meantime Wendy had arrived. She was in the resuscitation area and was standing next to Robert, often moving out of the way as various staff members attended to him. Whilst everything was well organised and going to plan, the room was busy, almost frenetic, as nurses, radiographers, resident and emergency department staff, anaesthetists and the surgical teams all intermingled: examining, talking, doing. I imagine it was an overwhelming scene for Wendy. We took Wendy aside and explained to her the problems and what we planned to do. I said we hoped to save and restore Robert's leg and warned her we might not be successful and would have to make decisions as we went, depending on how he responded and how viable his tissues were. She consented for us to proceed. Legally, we could have done so anyway, as it was life-saving treatment. On opening the abdomen the surgeon was confronted by a large amount of blood in the cavity. There was an extensive laceration to his liver, which the surgeon packed gently, but firmly, reducing a lot of the bleeding. The surgeon then discovered that a medium sized artery in the attachment of the small bowel had been torn and was bleeding briskly. It was possible to tie off this vessel leaving sufficient residual circulation for the bowel to remain viable. The spleen was bruised but intact and was not removed. Following this the bleeding in the abdomen appeared to be well controlled. The surgeon decided to leave the pack in the liver as Robert was still not well and further treatment of the liver laceration could be delayed quite safely. Injuries of this type often lead to swelling and pressure in the abdominal cavity and so the surgeon did not suture the abdominal wound but left it open, covered by a sterile plastic sheet and further dressings.

I then took over management of Robert's left leg. As we were preparing to do this my registrar reduced the dislocated right big toe, as it is very easy to ignore relatively minor injuries whilst pre-occupied with major ones, only to find later that these cause significant problems. We spent considerable time washing out the leg and removing dead skin and muscle and the contaminating gravel and dirt. The nerves to the foot were intact but stretched and exposed. We felt it probable they would not recover any useful function. One of the major blood vessels in the lower leg was torn and contracted, the other crushed and swollen. Four hours after the initial injury the foot was still pale and pulseless. Whilst Robert's blood pressure and pulse had stabilised, as most of the bleeding had been controlled during the abdominal surgery, his blood pressure was still low and the pulse rate high. The anaesthetist was concerned that he was still seriously ill. I paused to reflect and discuss our options. Our experience is that, in spite of all we have learnt and the techniques we can use to save a severely damaged limb, in this situation, the chances of Robert having a viable and usefully functioning lower leg and foot were very slim. If the leg is badly torn and crushed, as in Robert's case, there is also damage to all the small blood vessels and tissues, which significantly compromises recovery even if the blood supply to the large vessels is re-established. His leg was not going to survive for much longer without a blood supply and his condition remained poor and life threatening. We decided to amputate the leg through clearly viable tissue just above the knee.

How long a leg can survive without a blood supply depends on many factors. A fit young person can manage considerably longer than an elderly person with vascular disease and a very poor blood supply and chronically under-nourished tissues. We often use tourniquets in orthopaedic surgery to allow us to operate more quickly and safely in a bloodless field, where it is easier to see in tight and narrow spaces without blood getting in the way. This is particularly so when operating on bone with its extensive vascular marrow. Most of these operations can be done safely in less than two hours, but occasionally a tourniquet is left on longer. It is common practice to let down the tourniquet every hour or two for about five minutes to let the limb perfuse with fresh, oxygenated blood. In difficult and complex cases this may need to be done a number of times. At other times we accept the blood loss and difficulty to make sure the tissues remain viable.

Many surgeons recoil at the thought of amputating a limb, even removing a small toe feels intrinsically wrong. There is some primeval disquiet that we are doing wrong, no matter how rational the decision seems. The leg and foot were so severely damaged that we believed they were no longer viable and the breakdown products of dead tissue when released into the general body circulation are extremely toxic and life threatening. Leaving dead tissue also invites infection and gangrene. We decided to amputate his leg because we did not think it would survive in any useful way and leaving it on would significantly increase his risk of dying.

The thigh wound was packed and left open and covered with a dressing. Almost immediately the anaesthetist reported that Robert's condition had considerably improved, his pulse rate reduced and after further resuscitation and blood transfusion his blood pressure returned to normal. After two days in the Intensive Care department Robert's abdominal cavity was re-explored and the pack removed from the liver. The bleeding did not recommence. The abdominal wound was sutured and healed well. The leg wound was also explored and a small amount of residual dead muscle and skin removed and the wound again left open. Forty-eight hours later the amputation stump wound was clean and viable and was sutured and went on to heal well.

With the above-knee amputation Robert had a major sense of loss and a significant disability. After an extensive period of learning to use an above-knee artificial limb properly he was still unlikely to return to work functioning normally as an electrician and, whilst he would be able to retrain and continue working in some capacity, his life would never be as it was. Although he would adjust to it, and the modern prosthesis is very good, Robert would not fully return to the normal sports he loves, or play naturally and easily with his child as she grows up. He was quite likely to become depressed and, in association with a long period off work, this can cause significant problems in a marriage. Robert would regret the loss of his leg and wonder if it might not have been saved. Amid all of this he would be a man of unusual faith in surgeons if he did not question my judgment. Could and should I have saved his leg? Does he trust that I was competent and did my best to act in his best interest? I hope so, for if he does trust that I was acting to the best of my ability and understanding and treated him in his own best interests, as far as I could understand them, he will feel quite differently to the way he would feel if he believed I had been indifferent or careless of his interests and I had not done my utmost to help him.

We saved Robert's life, but that is what he expected us to try to do and hoped we would do. Yet we live in a world where we hear miraculous stories about surgeons saving limbs with microsurgery, hyperbaric oxygen and reattachments. The expectations of patients can be very high and sometimes unrealistic. Robert probably was not aware of the long and complex rehabilitation procedures associated with saving a severely injured limb. He would have needed extended periods in hospital with hard, painful, frustrating work to get his joints moving and build up his muscle strength. It takes at least two years to achieve maximum recovery. Even after such a long convalescence, for this type of injury the results are often far from satisfactory, especially if the foot is stiff and has limited sensation on the sole, as walking becomes very difficult and the foot is often cut when sharp objects are not felt and avoided. This often leads to infection and further damage to the skin and circulation. An early amputation with a good prosthesis can give a much better result. However, there is nothing as good as having your own functioning foot.

There is a complex interrelationship between my actions as an individual, as a surgeon, and as a member and a representative of a profession. The degree to which a patient might trust me may relate to my characteristics and reputation in all of these roles. Robert knew nothing of me and may not even remember seeing me prior to his surgery. Somebody probably proffered him a consent form to sign, but he would not have been able to make much sense of it. How can a patient know to trust me in my role as a professional and how useful are the ethics of the medical profession in protecting the public from breaches of trust?

Our concerns about trust are extensive. Can we trust the salesperson selling us our car and the mechanic who fixes it? What about the plumber who attends to our drainage charging a call-out fee and then by the hour? Are they working more slowly than they should? Are the problems the mechanic and plumber say they have found really there? Can we trust the clergy or teachers with the welfare of our children, or our teenagers with their own safety when one considers the ready availability of drugs and alcohol?

When we trust others we depend on their goodwill towards us, as I did, to my cost, with the girl on the train. This implies that ideally we must be able to recognise goodwill in others before we can truly trust them. We must be able to distinguish between the appearance of the self-interested compliance of a shopkeeper and the true goodwill of somebody we can reasonably trust to sell us the appropriate goods. Relying on somebody does not necessarily mean they will have goodwill towards us. By virtue of their occupation, shopkeepers might be relied on to find us things we wish to purchase, because they are trained to do so, and soldiers may stay at their post in spite of danger because they have a sense of duty or a greater fear of being court martialled if they do not. The surgeon operating on your leg may have no care for you whatsoever, but can still be relied on to do a good job because they have a professional commitment to their work or are interested in supplying a good service, as self-interest dictates they can in this way make a profit and do well in the world.

Nevertheless, it might be expected that somebody who willingly acts as a trustee would have some obligation to show goodwill, and to act from this goodwill, so that a truster can recognise that they are likely to be reasonably safe. It must be very confounding for a patient to find themselves in a situation where they need to trust a surgeon and they show no signs of goodwill, but rather appears disinterested, cold and unfeeling. We also need to be able to recognise that someone might in general have goodwill towards us, but not be inclined to act out of this goodwill, and be able to distinguish this from the person who has goodwill towards us and is motivated by that goodwill to act well towards us. For example, a surgeon may have goodwill towards me as a person, but not act out of this goodwill. They may like me as a person and find it pleasant to have me as a patient, yet recommend an operation that will expand a particular series of procedures they are doing, the results of which they wish to publish to enhance their career. The action is motivated by their desire to complete a series rather than to offer me the best treatment. They are not acting out of goodwill towards me.

Once we have given something that matters to us to the care of another and rely on their goodwill we become vulnerable to their choices and actions. Vulnerability in a trusting relationship is a particular sort of vulnerability. Once we depend on another's goodwill we are necessarily vulnerable to the limits of that goodwill and this vulnerability is different to that found in a formal contract. Contracts are drawn up to obviate the need for trust. Where it is quite clear exactly what each party expects from the other, as in a contract, the relationship suggests that one person is reasonably confident that the other will not take advantage of him. If one does in fact take advantage of another they have some redress, as they can claim compensation for any wrong. If a trusting relationship fails the truster often has no direct redress, except perhaps to take some form of revenge.

However, a contract might work to my disadvantage. If I were to insist on the letter of an agreement about some particular operative procedure and during that procedure it became apparent to my surgeon that continuing in the previously agreed manner would be to my disadvantage, it might be better for me if they contracted out. If my surgeon continued with our previously agreed, but in the light of their present knowledge inappropriate course of treatment, I might criticise them because they have made me even more vulnerable to damage. As this sort of situation happens not infrequently in medical practice, it thus follows that having a strictly contractual relationship between a patient and physician can turn to the patient's disadvantage. For instance, this can be a problem in childbirth where the woman has an agreement insisting on a 'natural birth' and changes her mind because of pain or safety concerns. Perhaps the best that can be made of a medical contract is that the doctor sticks to the spirit of an agreement. The nature of this spirit must be interpreted in any specific situation that may arise, as it arises, and therefore ultimately depends on the judgement of the doctor and their understanding of the best interests of the patient.

If we are able to trust, this allows others to perform a wide range of activities that cannot be managed with formal contracts, as no one can imagine or cover every situation or contingency. For instance, a surgeon may need to vary his technique during an abdominal operation because of unforeseen circumstances, a plumber might have to change to a different type of fitting because of a technical problem and a babysitter might need to call for assistance if a child becomes ill whilst the parents are away. Each of these people knows, or ought to know, that there is a limit to the decisions they can usually make without the truster's knowledge. Many decisions may ultimately need to be referred back to the truster for approval, although it is much easier for the householder and the baby's parents to assess and act than it is for a patient. Sometimes a trustee may have no choice but to act in circumstances in which they are ignorant of the values of the truster but would much rather have an idea of the truster's wishes. I would have preferred to have discussed the choices with Robert before amputating his leg, as a babysitter would prefer to pass important decisions back to the parents. A babysitter is different to the plumber and more like the surgeon in another respect, however, that is in the value of what they are looking after. Trust is something that assumes greater moment in our relationships with doctors and baby sitters than with other groups, given the greater significance and value of the things we are likely to cede to their control. If the trust fails the damage is greater.

Wrestling with the decision before we proceeded with Robert's amputation we paused and thought for a while. We were aware that our knowledge was incomplete and that our judgement could be at fault. Surgeons do have guidelines for the indications for amputation but they are inexact, as every situation is different. I had told Wendy of this possibility when she gave consent for the surgery but could have contacted her during the procedure to discuss it further. If she had been able to discuss the problems in detail with us, Wendy, I think, could not in the end have had the practical experience to make such a decision unaided. I did not contact her at the time as at that stage I believed that the ultimate decision was my responsibility as it was a life-saving measure and we needed to get on with it.

If we are able to trust others this also enhances the good of the community as a whole by allowing people to work together as teams. For example, when I was managing a sick patient, both the patient and I trusted various other doctors and nurses to perform their particular duties and allow each to make certain decisions with their own judgement. I trusted the anaesthetist to decide the type of anaesthetic they gave and a physician looking after the general health of a patient to act with the same autonomy. I trusted the nursing staff to contribute by making decisions within their own field without referring to me. This applies throughout the hospital environment, where many individuals and groups make their own decisions with the ultimate aim of acting coherently for the general benefit of the patients. No one person has the time or the expertise to double-check the actions of all of the individuals involved. This is not only a question of reducing complexity, but of cooperation so that a common goal can be reached.

Trust is valuable if it makes relationships easier. It allows the trustee to perform actions that they think are for the best without continually referring back to the truster. It saves both time and effort. This applies in many situations, but can particularly be applied to the doctor–patient relationship where the patient is often not in a good position to rationally assess information as it comes along. A surgeon cannot continually wake up a patient from an anaesthetic to ask for instructions, nor can they ask a patient about technical problems of which they have insufficient knowledge, or skills of which they have insufficient grasp. Ultimately, whether they trusted me or not, a patient sometimes had to trust my judgement. If they trusted me they may have been more comfortable about my judgement and actions.

There is some evidence that many people do wish to trust their doctor and use trust as a basis for the relationship. Deborah Lupton studied

330 patients in Sydney as she wanted to know whether the modern 'consumerist' movement had influenced the way people chose their doctor. She found that the majority of patients did not make a conscious effort to evaluate different doctors and they tended to pick one and then trust them. Lupton studied 60 lay people and 20 doctors. She found that there were some people who were rather 'consumerist' and 'shopped around'; that is, they sought out detailed information about the doctors they could access before making a decision about who to use. These patients were mainly the educated middle-class who were not very sick and who wanted a form of professional-to-professional relationship. There are also certain groups of people, like elite athletes for instance, who have networks of information and some knowledge of whom is considered, for example, to be the best surgeon to manage a particular problem. On the whole, older and less educated patients generally wanted to trust their doctor.

Lupton found that if patients became really sick then information, assessment and understanding became much less important to them and it was rare for somebody who was significantly ill to 'shop around'. Lupton comments:

> I think the relationship that people have with their doctor is almost a unique one. In any sort of relationship that we have with a professional or someone supplying us with goods or a commodity, even when you look at lawyers or accountants or dentists, you're still not putting yourself in their hands, you're not putting your life in their hands as you are with a doctor. In that situation, where really you're talking about matters of life and death, and you're talking about your own body, you're talking about doctors having access to your body, touching your body, cutting into your body in ways that other people don't have, then I think that's why it's so impossible to say, 'Well people should treat that person as if they were used car salespersons', because in that context trust is just a basic tenet of the relationship.

In discussing the good and bad stories that appear about doctors in the press, Lupton claims that people tend to remember the good stories, as they want to trust their doctor and it is in their interest not to remember the really bad stories. In some ways patients tend to filter out the really negative stories. They may notice but then forget them and think, 'Well my doctor's not like that'. Lupton concludes that, whilst consumer organisations do have a role to play in guiding people to make good choices, they tend not to take into account the idea that people do want to trust doctors and that patients may have a very emotional relationship with their doctor.

A number of conclusions can be developed from Lupton's study. Patients value the attentiveness and respect that a good doctor gives them and often consider this is the most important part of the relationship. Information sharing is also important and patients wish to be told what to expect by a caring doctor. This implies that it is up to the doctor to set the right expectations, as the patient will have trust in the fulfilment of these expectations. Patients expect their doctor to be responsible for the medical outcomes and in this to exhibit some autonomy. Nearly every doctor I have spoken to who has been ill will say that whilst they did consider knowledge and technical competence, they chose their own doctor as someone they knew would tell them what to expect and who would act in a caring way. They assumed the doctor would be responsible for the medical process and outcome.

Quite recently I was at a meeting of senior surgeons who were discussing various surgical approaches to the hip joint. This is a hot topic in the ranks of older community members, many of whom have arthritis and belong to golf, bowls and bridge clubs where they discuss these things. The introduction of a new approach from the front of the thigh, the 'anterior approach', has been claimed by some enthusiastic surgical advocates, many of them young, to be superior to the others. This approach has advantages and disadvantages and has yet to be properly assessed with long-term controlled trials. The senior surgeons concluded that were they faced with a hip operation, they would choose a surgeon they trusted and let them make the decision about the best approach. Sick doctors tend to act like other sick patients, although paradoxically, some can be wilful and excessively independent, sometimes to their own detriment. Doctors are very jealous of their independence and some do not like being advised, let alone told what to do, and can appear most unreasonable to others.

Lupton believes trust puts a significant onus on the doctor and that doctors feel the onus. She contends doctors in general have much the same idea about what constitutes being a good doctor and this includes having good communication and listening skills and being able to spend time with a patient, as well as having the required medical and technical expertise. On the whole, however, doctors welcome the consumerist approach as it makes them feel less like an idol and they express some relief that patients are becoming more willing and able to take some responsibility for their own health decisions.

Whilst it can properly be argued that the most important aspect of the doctor–patient relationship is about what is best for the patient and most satisfies the patient's autonomy, many physicians still cling strongly to the belief that their own autonomy needs protecting. An initial reaction to the idea of a doctor claiming some autonomy might be that this should be a very small part of a physician–patient relationship, as it is the doctor's role to help the patient. However, doctors can argue that one particular aspect of autonomy may be important, namely with decisions that sometimes need to be made by doctors as part of their role, such as when a patient, like Robert, is powerless. Whilst doctors can, and should, develop guidelines for the management of particular problems, it is often the case, as I illustrate in my example of Robert, that multiple factors are involved and likely outcomes are either unknown or can only be estimated as probabilities. Sometimes a doctor is presented with a number of possible actions and there is no clear guideline as to which is the best to take. The doctor can only come to the conclusion about the best action by reflection upon their broad knowledge and experience.

One of the cardinal features of a good doctor is their ability to make the right diagnosis in a complex situation and to apply it to the patient's particular personal and social situation. This can be described as 'clinical judgment', but what it constitutes is hard to clearly define. A decision based on clinical judgment may be difficult to defend if, in retrospect, it is shown to be wrong. The defence that a decision 'seemed right at the time' and was based on personal experience and insight is hard to justify to outsiders, particularly if they demand evidenced-based medicine. Clinicians, however, work in circumstances where the evidence is not always clear and each patient and circumstance is different. It is often not possible to practice on a basis of firm knowledge and established outcomes. If asked to describe what this good clinical judgement consists of, doctors might point to examples where a physician with good clinical judgement has consistently achieved what appears to be the best outcome over a period of time in a multitude of different difficult situations. This good judgment appears akin to what Aristotle called 'phronesis', or 'practical wisdom'.[19] The basis of much of the moral reasoning in this book goes back a long way to Aristotle, who many, including myself, regard as the greatest of all philosophers. He lived for 62 years in the fourth century BC, often in Athens. At other times he travelled widely and even did a stint teaching the young Alexander the Great. He studied and wrote on a wide number of topics, including biology, logic, politics, literary criticism and ethics. He had a remarkable ability to search out and analyse the essence of things.

Aristotle supplies strong theoretical support to a concept of clinical judgment that is based not just on knowledge, but also on skill and accumulated wisdom. Aristotle claimed that 'good' was not an abstract concept, but depended on what we wished to achieve. To become good at something we learn and practice certain 'virtues' (arête) and apply them in various ways depending on the circumstances. An Aristotelian 'virtue' is an attribute or skill that we use in order to do something well. The appropriate attribute depends on what we wish to achieve, whether it's playing music, sailing a ship or being a doctor. The attributes of a musician, for instance, are different to those of a sailor or a doctor. A musician needs to learn scales, develop pitch, tone and timing, and read music. A ship's captain needs knowledge of navigation, the weather and tides, and how to manage a crew and handle a ship. A doctor learns anatomy, pathology and the manifestation of disease and also needs to be able to communicate and have empathy and compassion. What makes someone a good musician is the ability to play an instrument to please his audience, a good sailor, the ability to cross the sea safely and in good time, and a doctor, to make a patient well.

Musicians learns their skills by practising. That is, they learn by 'doing'. The more they practice the better they get as musicians by using their skills well. Doctors and ship's captains are the same. As well as developing the required skills, all have to learn to apply them appropriately as it is one thing to have virtues and another to apply them well. For instance, courage is good in a soldier, but not if they foolishly take on all and endanger themselves and their comrades. Cowardice is bad in a soldier, but sometimes it is wise to withdraw. A soldier has to choose to behave somewhere between the two extremes of being foolhardy and cowardly. This is the mean. The mean, according to Aristotle, is never at a fixed point as sometimes a soldier needs to be courageous, other times prudent, and still other times, somewhere in between. Whichever action is appropriate depends on the circumstances and is always a matter of perception. Aristotle does not claim that every action consists of finding a mean, because some actions already have names that imply evil, such as spite, envy, theft and murder. In medicine we might include such actions as deceitfulness, sexual misconduct or not being trustworthy. Some things must always be wrong.

You become a good musician by being taught and practicing all the necessary skills and then by applying them to a particular work. Aristotle claimed that the actions of men become good or bad as a result of learning to act well or badly 'for if this were not so, there would have been no need of a teacher, but all men would have been born good or bad at that craft'. To act appropriately we also need to be able to understand how others think and feel and to empathise with, and be compassionate towards, their physical, emotional and spiritual needs. Whilst a musician applies a similar set of skills to all pieces of music, how and what they play may vary with the circumstances. That is a question of judgment. To play a happy dance at a funeral may be inappropriate, no matter the technical skills of the violinist, if the violinist is thought to lack sympathy for their audience. A happy dance may, at another funeral, be apposite if the mourners wish to celebrate a life lived well. Good judgment depends on the circumstances and is a matter of refined thought.

A person of practical wisdom is one who has learnt all the skills of their occupation and good living and has also developed the knowledge and sympathy required to apply these skills appropriately to particular situations. This is why empathy and compassion are moral virtues. To achieve this requires time, experience and reflection. Practical wisdom is not available to the immature, no matter what other skills and knowledge they have.

A person of practical wisdom is one who has learnt all the skills of their occupation and good living and has also developed the knowledge and sympathy required to apply these skills appropriately to particular situations. This is why empathy and compassion are moral virtues.

As the virtues of a violinist or a doctor are different, and have to be taught and practiced, the effectiveness of the use of these virtues, and their proper use, can only really be assessed by somebody else skilled in these virtues. The best judge of a particular subject is likely to be somebody who knows the subject, 'so the man who has been educated in a subject is a good judge of that subject'. Hence the only person who can truly appreciate the virtues required of a good lyre player is another lyre player. This does not mean that somebody else cannot assess the work of the lyre player, as we can all listen to the music and make a judgement about its beauty. Beauty is difficult to measure as the judgement of it is in the ear of the beholder and is a question of taste, although the skills required to achieve this beauty are specific and are not available to all.

People with practical skills make choices about the best action to take in particular circumstances. The captain of a sailing ship in a storm will have to constantly adjust their tack and the trim of the sails according to the direction and strength of the wind and the tides, all depending on the circumstances. Only a good ship's captain knows how to do this well. A passenger who arrives safely on the shore can acknowledge the skills of the captain but is not able to discover these skills simply by themselves. The art of being a good ship's captain is to be able to apply skills and knowledge well to the particular situation at hand.

Aristotle, whose father was a physician in the court of Macedonia, claimed that doctors are no exception to this, suggesting that the course to take in a complex situation is often a matter of judgement:

> In everything that is continuous and divisible it is possible to take more, less, or an equal amount. Thus a master of any art avoids excess and defect, but seeks the intermediate and chooses this: the intermediate not in the object but relative to us.

The right action to take in a particular circumstance is often a matter of perception and there is not an exact way of describing its worth. Virtues are tools to achieve a desired end and the virtues that one doctor would need to correct a broken ankle, such as manual technical skills, or treat a heart attack, such as having knowledge of the use of certain drugs, are different virtues. What matters is whether a doctor possesses and can apply the necessary virtues to a particular task in order to achieve a good outcome.

An approximate definition of clinical judgment is the ability of a doctor to discern the relevant features of a case, to estimate their importance and likely effect, to make reasonable decisions based on the knowledge they have and to apply these decisions well. These are the characteristics of a person of practical wisdom. Modern theory and research into the nature of how experts think suggests that experienced clinicians approach problem-solving in similar ways.[20] It is essential to have knowledge and clinical skills. With experience, clinicians develop a structure for dealing with complex or difficult cases and this process often appears to be unconscious and intuitive. The clinicians look for critical cues to the key features of the case they are dealing with and then delve into their memory for the relevant features of previous cases they have seen and produce a small set of possible hypotheses. They discriminate between the hypotheses and come up with the most likely diagnosis and most reasonable treatment. Sometimes this method is misleading and there is a danger of 'cognitive tunnel vision', that is, focusing on something that has had an impact in a past experience but is not relevant to the present problem. The whole process needs to be reviewed on a regular basis with corresponding self-criticism. In my orthopaedic and trauma practice we also regularly reviewed our decisions amongst our peers. Robert's case was fully discussed by the whole unit in our weekly meeting and my decisions reviewed in the light of the available literature on the management of similar problems and the combined experience of all those present.

So can we sit back, relax and confidently wait for the clever, wise doctors to make us better? Unfortunately not. There is increasing evidence that a well-programmed computer can often make better decisions than well-trained doctors. This has been shown in the diagnosis of chest pain, the interpretation of various cardiac tests, the diagnosis of appendicitis, the assessment by psychiatrists of the likelihood of parole violations by prisoners and many other instances. It is particularly valid in the issuing of medication prescriptions, where a computer is much more reliable in suggesting the right application and dosage of a particular drug and checking for and warning of the possible allergies and the likely adverse reactions with other drugs and conditions. Atul Gawande[21] has written a number of interesting, honest and open books reflecting on his personal experiences in training and practising as a surgeon and comments:

> Human beings are inconsistent: we are easily influenced by suggestion, the order in which we see things, recent experience, distractions, and the way in which information is framed. Second, human beings are not good at considering multiple factors. We tend to give some variables too much weight and wrongly ignore others. A good computer programme consistently and automatically gives each factor its appropriate weight.

There have been a number of scoring systems developed in attempts to rationalise the management of trauma. These list and attempt to weigh the impact of various aspects of a potential patient's condition, such as age, the time since injury and the site and degree of the injury. Useful guides, they are difficult to use reliably as they cannot assess complex problems. All injuries are different, many factors are involved, situations constantly change and many small decisions, which all add up, are made along the way.

The idea of sound clinical judgement is attractive but doctors have frailties, including bias and limited understanding, and do not always make rational decisions. Sometimes a well-programmed computer can be very helpful.

The idea that a patient may have to rely on the clinical judgement of a doctor is a difficulty in the doctor–patient relationship as the patient has no way of knowing just how good the clinician's judgement is. The only person who might know that is another similarly trained doctor or perhaps a well-designed computer algorithm. In my experience of patients who have had limb amputations in traumatic circumstances, one of the barriers to them accepting their amputation and coming to terms with it is a feeling of powerlessness, as they have not been entirely involved in the decision to perform the amputation. They may ask whether the amputation was really necessary and it is not always possible for the doctor to say honestly and with absolute certainty that it was, as the decision to amputate is a matter of judgement and not infrequently a judgement over which the surgeon himself anguishes in his uncertainty. If it is possible for Robert to believe that I made a decision in his best interest and did have an appropriate degree of clinical judgement, and applied my skills and knowledge well, then this may be a considerable help in him coming to terms with the shock of the amputation. This is more likely to happen if he believes that I have the characteristics of a trustworthy surgeon and if he does trust me. If he does not trust me he may always grieve that his limb was lost and believe it could have been saved.

We have seen that doctors can be unable to imagine the possibility that something could happen, even when they know of that possibility, and it is not uncommon for complex situations to exist where vital decisions are made without a patient being aware of them, or being able to understand them or to consent to them. Even in the best hands there is uncertainty and we may never know whether the correct decision was made. Patients may be vulnerable yet need to rely on the goodwill of the doctor as well as their knowledge and skills, and there are advantages in trusting in decisions that can be made expertly, simply and quickly. Sick patients want to, expect to be able to, and are prepared to trust doctors to look after their best interests, and the knowledge of this places a significant onus on the doctor. The idea of sound clinical judgement is attractive but doctors have frailties, including bias and limited understanding, and do not always make rational decisions. Sometimes a well-programmed computer can be very helpful.

Chapter Four: Rationality

Adrian and Brian are two soldiers[22] who go out on patrol and are alone together well away from observation. They come under fire from a single sniper and both know that they and their comrades back at base will be better off if they work together to kill the sniper. The sniper can only shoot at one at a time so if one of them quickly turns and runs he may escape but leave his partner at greater risk. No one will know if one runs off leaving the other to be killed. Adrian could easily run off and then go back to his unit and say that he had fought very hard alongside Brian but unfortunately Brian had been shot. Here are two people who are alone with each other, who know they will be consistently better off if they stand together, although it might be better for one to run, yet there is no obvious external constraint to hold them together. Any constraint must therefore come from within the relationship itself. Brian needs to be able to trust Adrian to stand firm and vice versa. For Brian, the crux of the situation is that Adrian, being human, is not completely reliable, as he has fears like anybody else, but Brian considers that Adrian has certain characteristics which will make him more likely than not to stand firm. One cannot imagine Brian willingly deciding to go on patrol with Adrian if he felt that he would run any time there was danger. Therefore Adrian has to have and be known to have certain characteristics that Brian values and these characteristics, apart from his strength and military skills, must mean that he can be trusted to behave in certain ways in certain situations. Brian, of course, may have no say in who his companion is. This decision may devolve to his superior officers. In a similar way a patient may have no choice but to trust a doctor in an institution so some responsibility must also devolve to his profession and the administration of the institution.

But what if the situation changes? What if the soldiers are outnumbered or outgunned? Might it not be better for them both to cut and run? In some situations one or both of the partners may have to make a decision.

What does Adrian do if Brian is injured? It might be better for him to stand and help Brian as they both might get out of a dangerous situation by standing together. However, it might be prudent for Adrian to realise that he is unlikely to live while saving Brian and so it would be better for him to run. Both Adrian and Brian have to make decisions as circumstances change and these decisions affect both themselves and their common good. Sometimes it's more valuable to look after our own interests, but only once it has become clear that acting together would be futile or counterproductive.

If Brian is attacked and falls and Adrian, quite prudently and correctly, decides to run, how will he be received when he goes back to his base? His fellow soldiers do not know what has happened and they have to make a judgement on Adrian's version of the story. They have to decide if he is telling the truth or if he is a coward and has run away and left Brian to perish. They cannot know the truth; all they can do is rely on what they know about Adrian and whether his personal attributes make him trustworthy and truthful. They can only know this through their observation of his past actions and their knowledge of his attitudes and values over a period of time.

Thus whilst we may, and often do, trust people without knowing them, we usually need to have some knowledge of how someone is likely to behave in the circumstances. This may come from knowing them well enough personally but often must come from our assessment of the role they play in society. We trust a stranger in a library in part from habit, but also from our knowledge of how they are likely to see themselves as a visitor to the library. Their likely motive for being in the library is to look at books and not to attack me. Thus my doctor, even as a stranger, is likely to behave in certain ways towards me because they are doctor and have learnt how to behave as one.

It is not sufficient that both of the soldiers are trustworthy, they both have to be able to trust each other. Brian's attitude to Adrian is as important as Adrian's is to him. If Brian thinks that Adrian will run away at the first sign of danger Brian will also run away, as he knows if he does not he will be in more danger than he was. Now it may be that Adrian is not trustworthy and Brian is right not to trust him. If that is the case Brian ought not to be out with Adrian in the first place. On the other hand it could be that Adrian is trustworthy but Brian is such a person that he is not able to trust him. If Brian has been persistently betrayed and doesn't trust anybody, having Brian out with Adrian would be a mistake, because as soon as there was danger it could be predicted that Brian would run away. Even though Brian might be trustworthy, if he cannot trust others he will be as useless and as dangerous as if he were not trustworthy. Thus it is an advantage to Adrian and his community if Brian is able to trust. We value both a trustworthy person and one who trusts wisely, and do not value either an untrustworthy or a non-trusting person.

Russell Hardin[23] writes an account of trust as 'essentially rational expectations about the mostly self-interested behaviour of the trusted'. Hardin claims a person should be considered trustworthy only when that person has an incentive to be trustworthy and is not surprised, and feels others also ought not to be surprised, if a trusted person becomes untrustworthy when that incentive goes. He claims that we should trust only when we can see that the person we are trusting has a commitment to their own gain from the trusting relationship and it follows that we can rationally trust doctors only if it is in their interest to be trustworthy. Hence it is not rational to trust anyone without having sufficient knowledge of that person's beliefs, needs and desires influencing their attitude towards us. This appears to preclude that we can rationally trust strangers, yet we seem to trust strangers all the time. Not only do we trust doctors we have never met before, we sometimes trust strangers in the street and used car salesmen even when we suspect we should not. Hardin argued that any trustworthy behaviour exhibited by medical practitioners is based on self-interest and anyone trusting them should realise this and only trust according to their own self-interest. Hardin[24] later modified his position to claim that we can learn to trust from past experiences and 'the best device for creating trust is to establish and support trustworthiness' so we should use certain devices to make people 'trustworthy', including contracts, social sanctions and institutional rules.

Martin Hollis[25] used game theory to assess whether two people, each acting in such a way as to maximise their own preferences, could achieve a goal that was maximally beneficial to both of them. He was unable to show that rational self-interest can achieve this and predicted that if individuals act only to maximise their own preferences they are never likely to maximise their goals, as they will always be forced to compete with or undermine other individuals. The only way for people, acting purely rationally, to achieve some form of progress and mutual satisfaction is to organise themselves into a sort of 'team which has common goals'. But that does not solve the problem of one team working against another. Because we will always be competing with each other, thinking in terms of rational self-interest tends to destroy trust.

The rational process, although it is a method of thinking based on the critical or logical development of ideas and actions from information, falters with the realisation that most of the information we consider 'factual' is a mere plausible assumption or value-laden assessment. Bertrand Russell[26] argued that the only reason that we really have for believing something like the sun will rise tomorrow is based on the observation that it has always done so in the past. There is always some doubt whether the sun will rise in the morning, although the more knowledge we have about the laws of motion and the movements of the planets and heavenly bodies, the more likely we are to feel confident about the sun rising. Russell argued that we are not able to prove that certain things must happen, but only reason in favour of the view that they are more likely than not to be fulfilled. As we extend our interest in expectations to the behaviour of people, we note that the probability of our expectations being fulfilled diminishes as more variables and uncertainties enter. The major stumbling block in rational thought remains the difficulty of ascertaining factual knowledge. Our attempts at rational thought must depend not on facts, but on the logical application of the best available credible information. This is not the same as true knowledge, but does depend on evidence and measurement to a greater or lesser extent. Excluding things like a mathematical or geometric argument that is based on a standard set of previously agreed rules, we can never be truly rational as we can only make best guesses using the information that is available to us at the time. Russell cautions us about relying on our experience and the expectation that the same succession of events will always follow. He gives an example of domestic animals expecting food when they see the person who usually feeds them, but

> We know that all these rather crude expectations of uniformity are liable to be misleading. The man who has fed the chicken everyday throughout its life at last wrings its neck instead, showing that more refined views as to the uniformity of nature would have been useful to the chicken.

If, as Russell argued, all our expectations of future events are based on inductive thinking from that which has happened in the past, we will be seriously disturbed if those expectations are unfounded because we have no other way of predicting the future and ordering our lives. According to Russell 'The most we can hope is that the oftener things are found together the more probable it becomes that they will be found together another time, and that, if they have been found together often enough, the probability will amount almost to a certainty. Probability is all we ought to seek'.

Peter Singer[27] discusses the dilemma that can be faced when each of us, individually, chooses what is in our own interest when dealing with others. In his opinion we are worse off than we would have been if we had each made a choice that was in our collective interest. Singer cites the well-known example of the 'Prisoner's Dilemma', in which two prisoners, unknown to each other, are given choices whether to confess or not. In essence, the outcome is theoretically best if both prisoners put the common good first, but as they don't know each other and probably will never see each other again, it is more likely that each will choose what is best for themselves, even though that result will not be as good as if they were able to work together for their common good. Singer comments:

> Without sanctions to back it up, an agreement is unable to bring two self-interested individuals to the outcome that is best for both of them, taking their interests

together. What has to be changed to reach this result is the assumption that the prisoners are motivated by self-interest alone.

Singer argued that a pair of altruistic prisoners was likely to come out of the situation better than a pair of self-interested prisoners, even from the point of view of self-interest. Altruistic behaviour, that is behaviour that benefits others at some initial cost to oneself and is motivated by the desire to help others, can work to the genuine advantage of both individuals. This seems possible only if both genuinely care more for each other than they do for themselves, an unlikely event if they are strangers or mere acquaintances although it is certainly possible in a loving, close friendly or family relationship. Singer notes that altruistic motivation is not the only way to achieve a happier solution. 'Another possibility is that the prisoners are conscientious, regarding it as morally wrong to inform on a fellow prisoner; or if they are able to make an agreement, they might believe they have a duty to keep their promises.' An alternative that Singer does not discuss is that the two prisoners have a strong commitment to trust and not betray each other.

In discussing the limits of self-interest the eighteenth-century Scottish philosopher David Hume wrote:[28]

> Your corn is ripe today; mine will be so tomorrow. 'Tis profitable for us both that I shou'd labour with you today and that you shou'd aid me to-morrow. I have no kindness for you, and know you have as little for me. I will not, therefore, take any pains upon your account; and shou'd I labour with you upon my own account, in expectation of a return, I know I should be disappointed, and that I should in vain depend upon your gratitude. Here then I leave you to labour alone: You treat me in the same manner. The seasons change; and both of us lose our harvests for want of mutual confidence and security.

Hume believed it is natural for man to behave selfishly but in doing a service to another he can foresee the service may be returned and can learn cooperative behaviour is helpful to all. The farmers learn that if the help is not reciprocated both are worse off. A significant difference between the prisoner's dilemma and the farmer's, is that the prisoner's dilemma only happens once in a lifetime, as the prisoners are unlikely to see each other again. The farmers have to live next to each other all the time and are able to develop a relationship of trust. Hume wrote that this practical application of self-interest does not 'entirely abolish the more general and noble intercourse of friendship and good offices'. He observed that it is quite possible for us to act, not just out of commercial interest, but because we have particular regard for certain people and work cooperatively without any prospect of advantage. Hume argued that we recognise and bind ourselves to the first or commercial form of cooperation, that of rational self-interest, by making and sticking to promises and so give each other signs that we are likely to stick to our promises. We are bound by promises and a man 'must never expect to be trusted anymore, if he refuse to perform what he promis'd'.

According to Hume, the expectation of a common benefit leads to a first obligation: to keep our promises. The second form of cooperation, that springing from regard for people, leads to a second obligation, in which we feel we have some moral obligation to keep our promises. The strength of these obligations, according to Hume, comes from the natural affection we have for each other, as 'all morality depends upon our sentiments'. Singer does not advocate that self-interest should be the only motivation for good human interaction as he acknowledges the warm feelings we have towards our friends and relatives and how we enjoy spending our time with them and cooperating with them. We form bonds with them that are an effective way of bringing about cooperation. Singer comments that although such pleasures and rational assessments may have evolved because they bring us benefits, our 'friendly feelings are no less genuine for that'.

Robert Axelrod[29] set up a game similar to the Prisoner's Dilemma, which was played multiple times with the same partner. The game was then played with multiple partners and Axelrod assessed what strategy achieved the best results for each individual. The best strategy was a relatively simple one called 'Tit for Tat'. This consisted of:

(a) On the first move, cooperate.

(b) On every subsequent move, do whatever the other player did on his or her previous move.

If one partner is cooperative and trustworthy then it is better to respond in the same manner, but if the partner is selfish and untrustworthy then it is best to respond uncooperatively on the next turn. Over a period of time those people who have cooperated and trusted each other perform better than those who do not cooperate or do not trust each other. If you are dealing with someone who is not trustworthy it is best, as soon you find this out, not to trust them and to respond in the manner in which they treated you. Even though it is good to be nice to each other, if we are constantly nice without reciprocation, then less-than-nice people will take advantage of us and our good nature. On this point Singer argues 'if there are no suckers, cheats do badly'. It is important to have strategies that disadvantage those who wish to take advantage of us and our good nature. If the less than nice do not cooperate or try to take us down then we should reply in kind. 'Being a sucker is not only bad for oneself but for everyone as it encourages deceitful behaviour.' In other game experiments[30] in which people can win money if they are generous to one another and if some individuals take advantage of this and accumulate more than their fair share, at a cost to the group as a whole, the disadvantaged majority will object to this. If the disadvantaged have a chance to financially penalise the miscreants they do so, even if this leads them to suffer some financial penalty themselves. If this activity is repeated, the selfish person may realise that they are likely to be punished for their behaviour and may learn to cooperate more. Thus in the short term the disadvantaged majority may initially lose out, while in the longer term punishing and attempting to re-educate an offender does pay off.

'Tit for tat' is remarkable for another reason. Russell Hardin presents a common view that we should not trust people until they have earned our trust. Tit for tat suggests that in a successful strategy we trust first and only distrust if that move fails. That this strategy works suggests that when we trust first up there must be a reasonably good chance that this will be reciprocated. If there was little chance that our goodwill would be returned, then we would soon give up trusting and would not be able to achieve things together. For Tit for Tat to be successful there also has to be a good chance that others will trust first as well. Tit for Tat implies we are taking something for granted about the positive behaviour of others. It appears to be in an individual's best interest, looking at the world rationally, to be both shrewdly trusting and genuinely trustworthy.

It appears to be in an individual's best interest, looking at the world rationally, to be both shrewdly trusting and genuinely trustworthy.

Annette Baier[31] describes trust as 'The phenomenon we are so familiar with that we scarcely notice its presence and variety'. She sees the idea of trust as pervasive and something we take for granted, though difficult to pin down and we may only notice trust when it has been broken. Baier expects strangers will not show her ill will and trusts strangers in the street or in a library not to harm or to interfere with her. The idea that a stranger might not show her, as an individual, ill will suggests her identity as an individual is important, even to a stranger. Baier's account of trust is not merely one of broad social expectations but something that individuals take into account as affecting them personally. This, of course, relies on other individuals in her community, and the community as a whole, accepting, acknowledging and honouring her individuality. Hegel argued that:

> Habit blinds us to that on which our whole existence depends. When we walk the streets at night in safety, it does not strike us that this might be otherwise. This habit of feeling safe has become second nature and we do not reflect on just how this is due solely to the working of special institutions. Common-place thinking often has the impression that force holds the state together, but in fact its only bond is the fundamental sense of order which everybody possesses.

We do not notice trust until it has broken down because we have not been conscious of the bonds that underpin our sense of order or the importance of the special institutions that create and support those bonds. Unfortunately, this sense of order has never been universal and has only been present in certain cohesive societies, such as those inhabited by Baier and Hegel. It can be very scary out alone at night.

Some societies have been able to develop quite complex relationships based on trust. Bruno Malinowsky[32] described the ritual passing on of objects such as necklaces and bracelets from one individual to another practised in the islands to the north and east of New Guinea. This is called The Kula Circle. Every man has one object in his hands at any given time but is obliged to continually pass the object onto another man, so that it will eventually move from one to another around a 'ring'. Malinowsky describes this practice, which is based in myth, backed by traditional law and carried out in accordance with definite rules, as a metaphor for a cooperative practice that is fixed and binds into partnership thousands of individuals. The partnership implies various mutual duties and privileges and symbolises a relationship that gives a basis to economic mechanisms, producing a specific form of credit that implies a high degree of mutual trust. The various groups of men meet occasionally and together reinforce their relationships. No man is able to keep an article for very long but each man has a large number of articles passing through his hands during his own lifetime. He enjoys temporary possession of each article, which he keeps in trust for a time. The Kula Circle allows the men to cement, by ritual, the ties necessary for mutual trust. While this trust does suggest a strong expectation of behaviour it also gives the individual responsibility to receive and pass on these symbols of trust. The Kula Circle acts as though to institutionalise the bonds between men by reinforcing a fundamental source of order. This idea might also help to explain the sense of ritual and 'dressing up' that Daniel[33] describes in the professions, as the ritual acts symbolise the commitment of the individual to the group. The external trappings and ritual of the professions reinforce Hegel's unconscious sense of order and is based on trust.

Axelrod reports four factors that tend to make Tit for Tat successful.

The first two factors are the avoidance of unnecessary conflict, by cooperating as long as the other player does, and clarity of behaviour so that the other player can adapt to your pattern of action. Importantly, the other two factors are provocability in the face of an uncalled-for defection by the other and forgiveness after responding to a provocation. Robert Trivers[34] suggests that if a cheater in a reciprocal relationship is found out, one way of their being able to re-enter a trusting relationship is to make some reparative gesture. Trivers also suggests that it is plausible 'That the emotion of guilt has been selected for in humans partly in order to motivate the cheater to compensate his misdeed and behave reciprocally in the future and thus to prevent the rupture of reciprocal relationships.' Axelrod says Tit for Tat is a very easy game to play because you do not really need to think rationally, you just have to follow simple rules. He also states that there is no need to assume trust between players, as the use of reciprocity can be enough to make defection unproductive and altruism is not needed as successful strategies can elicit cooperation even from an egoist. But you still have to trust the first time.

Trust is assumed as an unconscious recognition of the underlying bonds that have been developed out of habit, practice and probably some inherited characteristics. For this cooperation to be successful it must occur over a period of time and the players must have a large enough chance of meeting again so they do not discount the significance of their next meeting. Another requirement is to begin the game of Tit for Tat there must be some recognition by a number of individuals working together that they should use this technique. These last two requirements are met if we recognise Hegel's society of people working together, out of habit and with good upbringing, with a rational appreciation that what is good for each is entwined in what is good for all.

> What is of the most importance is that the law of reason should be shot through and through by the law of particular freedom and that my particular end should become identified with the universal end or otherwise the state is left in the air. The state is actual only when its members have a feeling of their own self-hood and it is

stable only when public and private ends are identical.

A trusting relationship may also depend on the rational assessment of the values of both parties. For example, Adrian discovers he has an infection after a sexual adventure and is very distressed and is not sure how to cope with life. He confides this knowledge to his friend Brian and asks him to keep it secret. Brian understands that Adrian has confided in him because they are friends and to help him cope with his emotional distress. Brian is aware of his special position as a friend and knows the distress that would be caused, both to Adrian and to the friendship, if he were to divulge the secret to anybody else. Subsequently Adrian establishes a sexual relationship with another individual, Clive, and tells Brian that he has no intention of telling Clive of his infection. Brian feels that he ought to tell Clive but knows that he is being trusted not to reveal the information.

The relationship between the young men fulfils all the necessary conditions for personal trust. Adrian has voluntarily given his friend the information, yet cannot be absolutely certain Brian will not divulge it so relies on Brian's goodwill and would be very upset if his friend divulged the information to another. Between the friends there is no ignorance, deceit or ill will and Adrian was not unduly reckless in divulging information like this to his friend, as he needed to speak to somebody about it, and who better than your best friend? However, Adrian is vulnerable if Brian believes that Clive should be aware of the situation. Brian is faced with a major dilemma in which he has to assess his own values, as his friendship and obligation to Adrian conflicts with his ideals of justice and an obligation he feels he has to Clive. When Adrian decides to trust Brian with his secret he is likely to be aware that such a situation might arise, as it is the sort of secret that, by its gravity, puts particular stresses on the trustee.

Before Adrian and Brian can enter into such a deeply trusting relationship they need to rationally consider, if their relationship is to be a meaningful one, two major things. The first is the facts of the situation as they appear to each and the second is the knowledge of the values each holds. Each will have to consider what is known and what is unknown about the other, and the unknown facts and values, both discoverable and not discoverable. Before Adrian can rationally trust Brian with his secret he needs to know what sort of a person Brian is, whether he has been shown to be trustworthy with secrets in the past and whether he understands the importance of the sort of secret Adrian might give to him. The more Adrian knows about Brian and the closer a friend he is to him the less risk he will take. But Adrian also needs to know about Brian's values. He needs to know the importance of this particular friendship to him, whether he values individual friendships over general considerations of justice, what he thinks of himself and how much he values being trustworthy.

Before Brian can rationally accept responsibility for sharing a deep secret with Adrian, and look after that secret, he has to know something about Adrian, about what sort of a person he is and whether he is worthy of support. What if Brian thinks Adrian is a very careless person whose secrets are not worth keeping? He also needs to know about which particular goods Adrian wishes to have cared for and the values he holds. He needs to be particularly aware of what having the infection means to Adrian and what having a close friend means to him. If Brian can see that keeping secrets safe is important to Adrian, he will weigh this more heavily than if he feels Adrian does not care too much about it. It may not be easy for Brian to fully understand Adrian's values but to make a decision in this situation he will need to find out as much as he can.

Adrian does not know what attitude Brian will take until Brian knows what the secret is. If Adrian does not check with him then Brian has not been given a choice about whether he is prepared to accept the responsibility of the secret. Brian may object to having been given the secret if he feels his commitment to Adrian is not strong enough to warrant taking on something that might be a great imposition on him. Brian might not think much of his friendship with Adrian at all so might prefer to say to him that he did not want responsibility for a secret of that magnitude. Brian might think their friendship is not sufficient to overcome any conflicts outside the friendship associated with this knowledge. Brian might consider that justice and taking care of the interests of the third party, Clive, are much more important than his friendship with Adrian. Therefore, Adrian ideally must allow Brian a choice about how much responsibility he wishes to accept and how much commitment he wishes to give. In certain friendships, such as between married couples or long-term close friends, this sort of commitment might be taken for granted, but in other friendships each needs to consider the other's feelings on the matter. The relationship between them can be significantly diminished if Adrian is reckless, in the sense that he does not sufficiently consider the goodwill and values that Brian holds and the degree of commitment he has to their friendship. One certainty is that if Brian does reveal the secret to Clive, Adrian will have a strong emotional reaction when he finds out.

If Adrian decides to trust his doctor with the information he faces a different situation to confiding in his friend. The doctor will probably not consider his relationship to the patient to be one of friendship and will not have a friend's same desire or motivation to keep the information confidential. The obligation will be that of professional confidentiality. This professional confidentiality will be tempered by the doctor's duties to other patients and they may weigh their duties to a third person more heavily than a friend would. Doctors are also under a legal obligation to the community. An example of the difficulty of confidentiality and a doctor's duty to others is the American *Tarasoff Case*.[35] In brief, a patient confided in his psychiatrist his intention to kill Tatania Tarasoff. The psychiatrist did not warn Tatania of this threat, on the basis of the importance of confidentiality in his relationship to the patient, but unfortunately the patient subsequently killed Tatania. A court found that whilst the protection of confidentiality is very important, this ought to yield when disclosure is essential to avert serious danger to others. The judges ruled that, 'The protective privilege ends when the public peril begins'. If the doctor–patient relationship depends on trust this relationship is complicated if it is known that a doctor can either invoke or be coerced by the legal system. If a psychiatrist has to warn his patients that he may break their trust then a patient may be less likely to trust him and this will inhibit their dialogue and probably reduce the chances of the patient being helped. Sometimes confidences may be justifiably breached, as Adrian's doctor could argue that he has a strong duty to inform Clive as part of his public and professional roles. The realisation of this might appease Adrian, yet it would not be surprising if he still felt betrayed, even though he was aware of the doctor's other duties. As I have argued, this supposes that the patient expects more than a contractual relationship with his doctor, otherwise they would have no reason to react emotionally to any breach of confidence.

Chapter Five: Autonomy

Many years ago an elderly lady consulted me because she had pain in her hip. After explaining the diagnosis I thoroughly discussed all her treatment options with her, including an assessment of a number of operations with a list of their relative advantages and possible complications. I advised her to consider the matter carefully and to decide what she would prefer to do. She said she understood the situation clearly and had no more questions to ask. The next week her niece, who was a nursing colleague, rang to tell me that her aunt had thought me a kind man, but had regretted my inability to come to a decision and had sought treatment elsewhere. She, I began to appreciate, had wanted me to be involved in the decision she had to make and to guide her in making this decision. This failure in communication came about directly as a result of my desire to take what I then perceived as an enlightened approach to our relationship and to openly embrace her autonomy, but I misunderstood what she wanted and needed from me and what autonomy meant to her. On reflection, I think she had trusted me and expected me to act in her best interests. She expected more from me than I would have expected from my stockbroker, who would present me with a list of possible stocks in which I might care to invest with a short discussion of the advantages and possible disadvantages. He emphasised that he was only giving advice and any written advice was accompanied by a disclaimer that he would take no responsibility for my decisions. The stockbroker appeared to act with appropriate propriety and I expected and wished for no more from him.

Some patients don't want much information, others have little choice, and others are given no real choice as they are not told what they need to know, even when it is available. George was a sixty-five-year-old man who was advised by his local doctor to have a Prostate Specific Antigen (PSA) blood test done. This test has been widely recommended as an indicator of the presence of prostate gland cancer and has been used as an indication for prostate biopsy and possible radical prostate surgery if cancer is found. For some years there has been growing disquiet , however, amongst the medical community concerning increasing evidence that radical surgery for prostate cancer probably only gives a small increase in survival times and that the surgery has significant complications, including incontinence and impotence. George, along with the majority of the normal population, was not aware of this disquiet and followed the advice of his local doctor to see a specialist urological surgeon when it was found his PSA was moderately raised. The surgeon advised a prostatic biopsy, which showed prostate cancer, and subsequently advised radical surgery. At no stage did the surgeon or the local doctor advise George that there was a strong body of opinion who would have advised against the surgery, especially at his age. George did not have sufficient information to allow him to make any sort of properly informed consent. He had the surgery, suffered significant confusion for some weeks after and still has significant cognitive impairment. His life has changed as he now has difficulty remembering names, appointments, birthdays and many other things that make life commodious. Ironically, the pathologist's report showed the tumour had not been completely removed and the operation did not achieve what it was meant to do.

The concept of informed consent enshrines a relatively simple idea, that patients are entitled to make their own decisions about medical treatments or procedures and should be given sufficient information on which to base these decisions. This information should be provided in a form and manner that helps patients understand the problem and the treatment options available that are appropriate to the patient's circumstances, personality, expectations, fears, beliefs, values and cultural background. Doctors should give advice without coercion and the patient should be free to accept or reject the advice. Also implicit in the relationship is that patients should be frank and honest in giving information about their own health and doctors should encourage them to do so.

Providing information to patients does not necessarily mean that they absorb and comprehend it. Ian Olver and others[36] investigated the impact of the design of their consent forms and information packages on patients receiving cytotoxic chemotherapy for cancer and found that most patients did not appear to understand the purpose of the information they were given and the consent forms they filled in. The patients had poor recall of the major facts about their treatment and older and less educated patients performed less well than the younger and better educated. Most patients had difficulty absorbing large amounts of information in a short time, although the patients themselves did not identify this as a problem as they may not have been aware of it. Olver believes that patients may overstate the goals and understate the risks of chemotherapy 'because health professionals frame the information in an optimistic light or because patients use denial'. Olver postulated that the full disclosure of side effects may increase the patient's anxiety and thus be undesirable. He suggested that disclosure be limited to the common or serious toxicities expected to affect a patient's decision to accept or reject treatment. This is a contentious issue and there is other evidence suggesting that full disclosure is not detrimental to patients in the long term, even if they have an initial increase in anxiety. [37]

Many professionals have problems communicating with people outside their profession. McCormack and others[38] asked fifty patients who were admitted to the orthopaedic department in the Mater Misericordiae Hospital, Dublin, to complete a questionnaire testing their knowledge of the orthopaedic terminology involving the procedures to which they were consenting. They found that the majority of the patients questioned were unsure of the meaning of what, to the surgeons, were such apparently simple terms as 'fracture reduction' or 'internal fixation' yet all of the patients questioned had signed consent forms for such procedures. One of the problems the author had in preparing the questionnaire was finding agreement amongst the surgeons themselves in defining some of the terms and phrases used. McCormack contends that, in a technically advanced specialty such as orthopaedics, many procedures are ill understood, even by other doctors, and he believes this probably holds true for all medical specialties. He suggested that truly informed consent would involve a prolonged process of patient education, perhaps to the extreme point that the only person who could really give informed consent about an orthopaedic procedure would be another orthopaedic surgeon.

Most, if not all, patients who appear to be giving consent are doing so to procedures they do not fully understand and because of this McCormack argues that there must be an element of trust involved in any process of giving consent. Manson and O'Neill[39] later came to similar conclusions with detailed and cogent arguments to support their position, but they present a version of trust that does not include an account of our emotions or human sympathy, something we shall see is very important to a full understanding of trust.

Most, if not all, patients who appear to be giving consent are doing so to procedures they do not fully understand.

Medicine, as a profession, has become fragmented with increasing specialisation and sub-specialisation and general practitioners now often do not see their patients on a regular basis and find it hard to get to know them well as people and subsequently have difficulty advising them about their options. With the increasing power of some pharmaceutical companies and health corporations and the proliferation of products and technical procedures, extending from drugs and equipment to complex surgical techniques, intensive care units, medical devices and instrumentation, comes the tendency for patient care to become secondary to other interests, such as the pursuit of profit or the reduction of costs. There is also a tendency for patients to expect, and sometimes demand, the latest high technology and this is matched by doctors being fascinated with this technology and being keen to use it. Both patients and doctors are contributing to the difficulty doctors have in maintaining their caring skills, which Merrilyn Walton[40] writes they 'get from talking and listening to patients'.

Walton believes the best way doctors can work to achieve the best for their patients is for trust to be a basis for the relationship. Unfortunately, she claims: 'we are constantly reminded of the importance of trust, not by reports of doctors adhering to principles of beneficence, but their failure to promote trust'. If interests such as money and power dictate patient care, trust will disappear. If this happens then, as Francis Fukuyama[41] claims,

> People who do not trust one another will end up cooperating only under a system of formal rules and regulations, which have to be negotiated, agreed to, litigated, and enforced, sometimes by coercive means.

Whilst patients may need to feel that they are making the choices, it may be that the vital choice patients have to make is not necessarily which treatment they may have, but which doctor they will have to advise and help them. In this context it may be more important to ask the question 'whom shall I trust?' rather than 'what shall I do?' This may be easier said than done, as often patients do not have much, or any, say in who looks after them.

A patient's autonomy can be easily diminished. Patients are often ill, frightened, confused, unconscious, demented or in many other ways powerless and not able to rationally control their plight. They are not always helped and advised by loving family and friends. The professional carers may be the only ones who are in a position to help and they may have, to the best of their ability, to imagine the patient's needs and best interests. Professionals, such as doctors, lawyers, dentists and accountants often have power over others because of their knowledge or expertise and this power can be harmful if it is exercised incompetently or thoughtlessly. This is an important aspect of professionalism because the professions claim some right to control their own work and standards, thus allowing them some socially recognised autonomy. Autonomy is central to the idea of a profession and carries with it an obligation to use it well in the public's interest. In order to deserve this level of autonomy, a profession must meet standards of ethical as well as technical competence and for this reason most professions have codes of ethics to delineate the standards their members are expected to uphold. Even though ethical codes reflect a profession's implicit promise to society to uphold standards of technical and moral competence, most of these codes are rather general and often not particularly helpful when applied to unique dilemmas. Ethical codes are guides to behaviour but are not able to advise the correct behaviour in specific circumstances nor do they give a patient much guidance as to how an individual or institution ought to advise upon or manage their own particular problem.

Many clinicians consider that true patient autonomy is almost always an illusion. Even an educated, alert patient is often not allowed to determine their own treatment, but merely to refuse or accept that which is offered to them. Patients can rarely successfully demand treatment that is either not readily available or which the carer does not wish to offer. The idea of informed consent is now structured so that the patient has the formal responsibility for their treatment transferred to them, even though they may at the same time feel quite powerless. The present structure of the many treatment consent forms is an excellent example of this, as the modern consent form is designed to protect the system and the doctor from being sued, rather than look after the best interests of the patient.

> *The idea of informed consent is now structured so that the patient has the formal responsibility for their treatment transferred to them, even though they may at the same time feel quite powerless.*

George was not given sufficient information to allow him to make an informed choice about his prostate operation. We all fear cancer, and the idea that a surgeon can cut a growth out and cure us is appealing and often justified. It would have appeared to George that it was as simple as that and he discounted the possibility of serious complications and had no hesitation in having the surgery as he thought the operation would save his life. However, the situation is not as simple as it first appeared. The evidence from controlled surgical trials is that surgery only marginally increases longevity in prostate cancer and then only after many years. Many experts now do not recommend surgery after the age of 65 and some do not recommend it at all. If it is to be done it may be only reasonable for younger men and then have to be carefully considered due to its not insignificant complications. George trusted his doctors but his autonomy was not truly honoured, and I see this as a betrayal.

Recent changes in the law concerning informed consent have emphasised the increasing importance judges, reflecting the society in which they live, have given to patient autonomy. The emphasis in legal judgments have gradually changed to reflect the circumstances of particular individuals and there is little doubt that the average patient is much better informed today than they were even a few years ago. There are problems with informed decision making, particularly in cases where people are diagnosed as mentally ill or intellectually disabled, but many people believe that the average patient can be sufficiently well informed to be able to make their decisions autonomously. Yet if each doctor must decide for each patient on each occasion, selecting information appropriate to the patient's circumstances, personality, expectations, fears, beliefs, values and cultural background, this appears to be asking a lot of doctors. Every person is a complex mix of these factors and it is not always clear, even to our own selves, where our particular interests lie.

It is probably best for patients to be given a clear, understandable explanation of the important and major complications of any treatment rather than a comprehensive review of all of them, along with a legal requirement to provide information that would, as held by an important Australian High Court decision in 1992 (*Rogers* v. *Whitaker*),[42] 'be reasonably required by a person in the position of the patient'. Mrs Whitaker had had a penetrating injury to her right eye as a child and, nearly forty years later, was referred by her general practitioner to an ophthalmic surgeon, Dr Rogers. Dr Rogers hoped to improve the cosmetic appearance of the badly damaged eye and possibly to restore some useful sight. He did not warn her of the remote risk (found to be about 1 in 14,000) of sympathetic ophthalmia, a complication she tragically suffered, thus losing sight in her good eye. Sympathetic ophthalmia is a condition in which an operation on one eye can cause blindness in the other, normal, eye. Mrs Whitaker lost the sight of her good eye, thus becoming almost totally blind. The High Court placed considerable emphasis on her 'incessant questioning' about the procedure and its complications, although she had not asked a specific question about possible damage to her good eye as she had not thought of that possibility.

Mrs Whitaker successfully sued Dr Rogers for negligence. The court accepted that Mrs Whitaker would not have undergone the surgery had she been advised of the risk of sympathetic ophthalmia and decided that a medical practitioner has a duty to warn a patient of a material risk inherent in any proposed procedure or treatment. The judges held that:

> A risk is material if, in the circumstances of the particular case, a reasonable person in the patient's position, if warned of the risk, would be likely to attach significance to it or if the medical practitioner is or should reasonably be aware that the particular patient, if warned of the risk, would be likely to attach significance to it.

It may not be immediately obvious that the difficulty between Dr Rogers and Mrs Whitaker was one of trust, or loss of trust. Mrs Whitaker needed to decide whether to have an operation on an eye that had troubled her for many years. She had managed her life reasonably well up until that time and any decision she made about the operation required her to balance the advantages of having some improvement in the look and function of her eye against the disadvantages of having surgery. In order to make that decision she needed all the information that was relevant to her. Dr Rogers withheld some information that Mrs Whitaker later believed would have, if she had possessed it, persuaded her not to have the operation. Mrs Whitaker argued that she could reasonably expect him to give her information relevant to her, so that she could make a decision based on her own values. Dr Rogers did not think the information was relevant to Mrs Whitaker and it is likely that he could rightly claim that he did not knowingly or deliberately mislead her. Dr Rogers substituted his judgement for Mrs Whitaker's judgement about the relevance of this information. Dr Rogers may have argued that it was not possible for him to know all of Mrs Whitaker's values, but the High Court reasoned that he should have been aware that the possibility of her going blind, even if remote, was relevant to her.

It is a reasonable argument that no one can completely know what another person's interests really are. In support of his view that trust in a professional relationship is not a valid concept, Robert Veatch[43], argued that:

> To the extent that it is impossible for professionals, (1) to know what the interests of clients are, (2) to present value-free facts and behaviour options, and (3) to determine a definitive set of virtues for a particular profession, then I am forced to the conclusion that professionals ought not to be trusted.

On the other hand, Manson and O'Neill suggest that the way we come to trust is primarily about assessing what others say or do and whether this fits in to how we see the world. Whilst we can get better at assessing others and learn to trust more intelligently, and get better at refusing to trust, it is not possible to know everything about another and all the circumstances. Manson and O'Neill believe an obligation to communicate, rather than to disclose, should be considered and the quality of this communication assessed. For a patient, doing without trust is impossible.

For a patient, doing without trust is impossible.

It is not possible to know the full interests of a patient, as it is probably not possible to fully know what anyone's short- and long-term interests are. Indeed, each of us do not seem able to fully and consistently understand and apply our own interests. However, it is usually possible to have some idea of the sort of interests a patient might have. A patient should be able to trust a surgeon with the idea that when he has a broken arm, which is clearly crooked and painful, it is in his interests for him to straighten it out and hold it still. A fit middle-aged man with a family, who has every other reason to live, if he is having a heart attack and fears he might die, should be able to trust a cardiologist to realise that he may wish to have treatment for this heart attack and it is not his bunions or wrist watch that need fixing. It would surely be that if Robert Veatch passed me on the side of the road and noted that one of the tyres of my car was flat it would occur to him that I might like help to fix it. He would not need to know all my enduring values, only that I would wish to go on with my journey, wherever that may lead.

Trust in medicine spans a wide spectrum from that between individuals in a single doctor–patient relationship, to multiple and complex interactions between a patient and hospital staff. Veatch could argue that I would not be able to define a good outcome for a stranger with a broken ankle, but that is something I could ask them. I could have some understanding that they might wish to have it corrected and be freed from pain and to be able to walk well afterwards, as those are things anybody can understand. I would not need to know all their dreams and aspirations and I can imagine any fear of surgery they might have. It would also be possible for me to understand that if it was someone's elderly mother, who was perhaps demented and towards the end of her life, who broke her ankle, she may not want to have any major reconstruction of her ankle but simply be made comfortable. In this situation I might need other fundamental virtues, like empathy and compassion, even though these are not specific professional virtues.

So, whilst it is indeed impossible for me to know every interest of a patient, or to produce value-free facts that the patient can understand, and for me to be able to explicate in detail all the virtues I might or might not possess, it is nevertheless possible for me to communicate a general understanding of these in the particular circumstances in which a patient and I might find ourselves. Whilst I disagree with Veatch that his criteria exclude the possibility of trusting a doctor, his argument does show that it may be difficult to judge in a particular case what constitutes the right action. This is particularly so if one considers the totality of the patient's situation and their complex enduring values and the doctor's role in interpreting these. I would conclude from Veatch's argument that there is a need for some sort of trust or else we will be frozen into inaction, as no one will ever have enough knowledge to make a decision.

Thus the High Court of Australia might be asking too much of doctors if it expects them always to know enough about each individual patient to be able to make judgements about what that patient needs to know and how they should present this information so that both the doctor and the patient have the same understanding of it. In this sense and at this level I would agree with Veatch that it is impossible, although it is something worth aiming for. But that is not to say that someone like Dr Rogers would not have been able to communicate with Mrs Whitaker about the possibility she might go blind. None of us would have much difficulty in being able to understand what it would be like for her to be blind, nor would she have any difficulty understanding what Dr Rogers meant if he told her that she might go blind. Of course, people have trouble estimating probabilities, as to some 1 in 14,000, the estimated odds against getting sympathetic ophthalmia, would be long odds, to others they would be short. We are able to understand things we can commonly imagine applying to ourselves and to others. It is difficult for any of us to enter into the more complex world of the overall totality of values and fears that people have and what their lives mean to them.

For every patient there must be a preferred position between receiving no information at all and all the information that is possibly available. The nature of this position will depend on the particular patient at a particular time. Knowing how much to tell a patient will depend on the circumstances and will fall between the extremes of telling the patient everything possible and telling them nothing at all. As Aristotle implies, some things, like deceit or lying, must be considered bad in themselves. To knowingly not give a patient information that is relevant to them or to give information that is incomplete or in a form that is difficult for them to comprehend, can be seen as bad in itself. Thus the decision to not give George all the relevant information about his prostate cancer was bad in itself. The burden of proof, if information is to be withheld for the supposed benefit of the patient, rests with the doctor and they should be prepared to present this proof to an outside authority, whether it be a court or a surrogate. Unfortunately, whilst Mrs Whitaker challenged the actions of Dr Rogers in the courts, it was not till after she was blinded that such a burden of proof was negotiated.

What would I advise the elderly woman with a painful hip now? I would tell her my diagnosis and summarise the advantages, disadvantages and the common and significant, even if rare, complications of the various treatment options, including non-surgical therapy. I would ask her if she had any particular concerns or questions and how she felt about the options. I would then advise her what I think she should do in her circumstances and suggest she take time to think about it. I would give her any patient pamphlets or other information that I had for her to read at home. Using this approach, my experience has been most patients decided then and there, and it was usually what I had recommended. Others needed more time for further thought or consultation and occasionally one left, never to be seen or heard of again.

Chapter Six: Respect for the Individual

Ron had severe arthritis in his hip and needed a total hip replacement. He understood the advantages and disadvantages of the surgery and felt he had sufficient information to make an informed decision to go ahead. Ron was happily married and loved his three young grandchildren and was distressed that he could no longer live a good life and play actively with the children. There were problems, however: he was a Jehovah's Witness and would not consent to a blood transfusion if it were required during the surgery. Through my own experience I had learnt that it was quite possible to do this type of surgery without a blood transfusion although it increased the risks if something went wrong. But Ron had a complex problem, as his hip socket had worn away so there was not enough bone to support the proposed new artificial socket and he required extra, more difficult and dangerous surgery to counter this. This meant that the need for transfusion was much more likely and the risks of complications and death greater than usual. Ron was still prepared to take the risk. The risk of death after conventional hip replacement is now down to about 0.3%, acceptable to most patients in severe pain, but I was unable to say how much higher Ron's risk was, except it was significantly greater. He also had an increased risk of complications such as infection, wound breakdown and nerve damage because of the longer, more difficult procedure.

I have had, and listened to, many conversations about Jehovah's Witnesses and their attitude to blood transfusion. They believe fervently that accepting blood from another, and even in some cases stored blood from themselves, is against God's will and will lead to eternal damnation. There is to some people a fate worse than death. They also fear banishment from their community. My attitude was to accept their belief and do my best to work within their self-imposed restrictions. Many people, however, consider their beliefs as irrational and claim they should be discounted. This particularly applies if their beliefs affect others, such as their children.

Immanuel Kant[44], the eighteenth century German philosopher, criticised his Scottish contemporary David Hume for allowing what Kant believed were dangerous sympathies and emotions to influence his moral thinking. Kant believed our emotions are far too likely to cloud our judgment to allow them to be used as a basis for good decision-making. Kant stressed the uniqueness of the rational human individual and argued that no human should be treated as a means to an end, but as something intrinsically valuable in himself. The rational human individual is the critical factor in Kant's moral thinking. All rational individuals who meet with like rational minds will produce a universal source of morality, as they must if they are thinking rationally together, and will develop certain principles of action that should be universally applied.

Kant is difficult to understand and explain. He believed that moral decisions could, and should, be made independently of our emotions and desires. A group of people who think rationally could, and would, agree on certain principles, regardless of their personal circumstances, that is 'a priori' – before knowing the facts. They would do this because they were rational and, if acting rationally, they must come to the same conclusions in the same situation. A group of rational subjects would all agree on certain principles of action and apply them at all times to all their actions, regardless of their personal circumstances. A rational person in this community would accept that these 'categorical imperatives' apply to themselves and all others. This is called Universalisation.

Kant's main maxims:

> Always treat others as ends in themselves (and not as a means to an end).

You must not use people for your own purposes but accept and honour their distinct and rational selves. Our modern ideas of autonomy come from this.

*Act only on that maxim which you can at the same time
will to be a universal law.*

If you decide to do something you must be able to agree that everybody
else should do it too. Hence the idea of universalisation.

*Act as a member of a community of like rational minds
(Realm of minds or Kingdom of Ends).*

Act as a rational member of society for reasons that every other person, if
acting rationally, must support. If every member of the community acts
rationally, given the same circumstances they will all come to the same
conclusion. This is the 'categorical imperative'. Examples of categorical
imperatives are that you should never kill, tell lies or break promises.

However, universal principles are often difficult to apply to individual
situations. Kant argued, for instance, that a community of rational
minds would have an imperative to never lie or break promises, but we
can all think of situations where it would appear appropriate to do both.
Kant answered this objection by saying you can never know what the
consequences of your actions will be and in the long run you will be worse
off if you do not follow these imperatives.

If, for a Kantian, autonomy is vital in the application of the Kingdom
of Ends, to treat a patient with respect is to treat them as if they were
using their reason and acting rationally within their circumstances and
beliefs. 'Even in a case where someone evidently is wrong or mistaken, we
ought to suppose he must have what he takes to be good reasons for what
he believes or what he does'.[45] This attitude is something we owe to the
patient, which the patient cannot forfeit. Kant claimed:

> Here upon is founded a duty to respect man even in the
> logical use of his reason: not to censure someone's errors
> under the name of absurdity, inept judgement and the
> like, but rather to suppose that in such an inept judgement
> there must be something true, and to seek it out.[46]

Patients are to decide for themselves what they think and choose to do. Poor judgement does not disqualify anyone for citizenship in the Kingdom of Ends. This kingdom is 'a systematic union of different rational beings through common laws'. A rational being is both a member and a sovereign of the realm as they are subject to the laws as well as being authors of them. This means there cannot be a good reason for taking a decision out of someone else's hands for 'reason depends on this freedom for its very existence'.[47] It is the patient's prerogative as a rational being to have a share in determining their destiny. Any attempt to control the actions and reactions of another by any means except an appeal to reason treats them as a mere means. If you make a straightforward appeal to the reason of another person your responsibility ends there and the other's responsibility begins. Robert Young[48], discussing such a rigid view, claims that whilst rationality is required for autonomy, as an autonomous person would make valid deductions from the available information, such a person acting autonomously would not be subject to unthinking submission to authority or acceptance of superstition and prejudice. Yet there seems no reason why life's choices have to appear rational to others, as one can choose a dissipated life, smoke cigarettes or choose a particular extreme religious sect and still claim to have a valid life-plan. The actions of a Jehovah's Witness in refusing a blood transfusion may seem illogical to some but are quite rational within the context of the Witness's belief that the Bible, to which they are committed, absolutely forbids this.

A definition of rationality must be something like the critical assessment of that which can reasonably be assumed to be a stable and plausible basis for argument. Yet if we are to respect patient autonomy then we must accept certain patients, who may appear to be acting in a most irrational fashion to us, may be acting quite prudently, sensibly and consistently with good reason within the assumptions that spring from the way they see the world. Ron's decision effected a wide range of other people. If he were to die his grandchildren would lose their loving grandfather and as they grew older may wonder why he had not considered them in his decision. His wife's attitude would depend on her beliefs and commitment to the faith. What is less understood is the responsibility he placed on me and the rest of my team. I have, in my younger days as a trauma surgeon, tried helplessly to save young people bleeding to death from abdominal trauma, desperately trying to stem bleeding from multiple areas, failing, and seeing them slip away and die. Even for a surgeon, that is not easy. Once, in Papua New Guinea, I remember a young patient dying in such a way. As we had limited help and space we covered his body and moved him to the side of the operating theatre as we went on to treat his friend, who we were fortunately able to save. In elective surgery, where a choice has been made to operate or not, such a situation is much more difficult and stressful. If Ron were to die in such circumstances it would take me a while to recover, if I ever really fully could. Other colleagues are also involved. My anaesthetist had similar feelings, which were complicated by his loyalty to me and trust in my judgment, as we had worked together for many years. He could have refused to give the anaesthetic but chose not to. The nursing staff and many others were also intimately involved and no less likely to be affected. They were also loyal to me. If Ron had died I would have had to break the news to his wife, suffer the inevitable criticism of others and then face the Coroner's Court to explain what happened. No amount of Aristotelian virtue theory would have saved me from that. Fortunately, after a great deal of care from all involved and a few anxious moments, Ron survived and went on to do well.

Ron trusted me with more than the usual person requiring a hip replacement does. Our legal position was quite clear, as Ron consented to the surgery and we documented that under no circumstances was he to be given blood or blood products. An adult person of sound mind is entitled to refuse treatment even if they will die without it. If I gave him blood this would constitute an assault. As well as the extra risks involved in the surgery, he also trusted me to allow him to die if something went wrong, and I accepted his trust. I had made a serious decision as well as he and had to accept the consequences. I can imagine the scene if he was bleeding profusely, we were having difficulty controlling it and I said he was not to the have the large blood transfusion we would have given in normal circumstances. The tension would mount as we struggled to staunch the flow and his pulse rate went up and became feeble and his blood pressure dropped to dangerous levels. We all would have thought that we were not doing everything possible to save him and be sorely tempted to break his trust, regardless of our legal duty. I had found it difficult in the past to watch a patient bleed to death in spite of my best efforts to save him, but this time I would be part of the decision that would lead to it. Around me were caring people who had not been involved in the decision but who would also suffer. If I had ordered a blood transfusion and he had survived I do not know exactly what Ron's reaction would have been, but if his beliefs were sincerely held, as I had no real doubt they were, he would have felt, at the least, grievously betrayed.

The tension would mount as we struggled to staunch the flow and his pulse rate went up and became feeble and his blood pressure dropped to dangerous levels. We all would have thought that we were not doing everything possible to save him and be sorely tempted to break his trust, regardless of our legal duty. I had found it difficult in the past to watch a patient bleed to death in spite of my best efforts to save him, but this time I would be part of the decision that would lead to it. Around me were caring people who had not been involved in the decision but who would also suffer.

Another criticism of the process of informed decision-making in medicine is that, even should patients intellectually understand the idea of a complication and be able to list common complications in a questionnaire, they may not necessarily be able to understand what it would be like to have the complication. It is one thing to know that you may have a complication and another to know what it is to suffer from it. Over the years I have seen most of the complications of total hip replacement and recognise the severe distress they may cause patients and often, to a lesser extent, the surgeon. One of the major complications of total hip replacement is deep infection in the wound, which can sometimes lead to a chronically painful joint and the need for multiple operations, extensive antibiotic use and the risk of total failure, leaving the patient severely disabled. I have seen patients who have had to have a leg amputated and painful, protracted treatment following chronic infection.

Douglas had a chronically infected open ulcer on his leg as well as severe arthritis in his hip. These ulcers usually occur due to poor circulation of the blood and sometimes take a considerable time to heal. Unfortunately, they harbour bacteria, which may spread to other parts of the body. This is particularly likely to happen if there has been a fresh wound and foreign material in the body, such as following a total hip replacement. The joint replacement may become infected and lead to severe complications and sometimes death. It is therefore important that all ulcers are healed and there is no sign of infection in the body before we proceed.

I explained to Douglas the difficulties and dangers of proceeding with surgery in such circumstances. He said 'I understand this and I know that I could get the complication of infection, but nevertheless I want you to do the operation because I am having so much pain in my hip and I will accept the risk'. As much as it is possible on a general definition of consent I would think it is likely that in this situation he was legally making an 'informed' decision. He knew the hip could be infected and what that could mean, but was ready to take that risk because he believed he was in sufficient pain to warrant the risk. I refused to do the operation until the ulcer was well healed. I did this on the grounds that I did not believe that Douglas fully appreciated what it was like to have an infection in a joint replacement and therefore he was not making a truly informed decision. Also, I did not wish him to have this complication for my own reasons: managing such a patient is time consuming and stressful and I did not want my operative infection rate any higher than it needed to be. In this situation legally I can refuse to operate. In an emergency situation I am obliged to help to the best of my ability, or if a patient is unhappy or disadvantaged by my refusal in a non-urgent situation, I am obliged to arrange further opinions and help.

By such action I risk being called 'paternalistic', but I believe I have a responsibility not to unduly place a patient at risk. I also have my own integrity and reputation to consider, including doing what I believe is wrong. Douglas trusted me in one way, but not in another, when he requested I should operate with such doubts in my own mind, as he was asking me to betray my own integrity. On other occasions I refused to operate on patients who requested it, usually because I did not believe an operation would help. There is no legal obligation on me to use treatment that I believe, with good grounds, to be futile.

It was not until I juxtaposed my account of Ron's situation and my decision to operate, with my decision to override Douglas, that I realised my position appeared contradictory. With one I took the risk of a man dying, with the other the risk of a deep infection. With one I acknowledged his Kantian autonomy, with the other I did not, claiming he lacked imagination. Both times I sincerely believed I was making a good decision. One reason I use to justify my decision was that Ron had an unshakable belief, fundamental to the way he saw his life, that I felt I must honour. Whereas an infected ulcer, whilst it might take many months of intensive treatment to resolve, is a potentially reversible, practical medical problem. I saw my role quite differently in each situation. I thought that Ron was making the decision and I was agreeing to co-operate fully with it, whilst in the other situation I was making the decision and forcing the patient to go along with it, although he could always opt out and seek treatment elsewhere.

Justin Oakley[49] argues that when we consider what counts as informed consent, in the context of other important ventures with uncertain consequences, informed consent does not necessarily require having complete information about one's future emotional state. To illustrate this, he considers a marriage contract, which we would accept could be entered into autonomously, even if later a person was left with enduring feelings of depression, loss and regret. He claims that these later feelings, and the earlier ignorance of their strength and meaning, do not undermine the autonomy of the original decision. He also argues that unforeseen post-operative depression, for instance, does not in itself show that the patient's original consent to undergo the operation was inadequately informed or non-autonomous. What is required for autonomous decision-making is not knowledge of the actual outcomes, but an adequate appreciation of the risks involved. Autonomous decision-making and informed consent seem compatible with a degree of uncertainty about the consequences, emotional or otherwise, of what we are deciding on or consenting to. It is our general experience that we can regret decisions we have made, and wish we had never made them, yet still take full responsibility for those decisions as we went into them, as it were, with our eyes open. The consequences of our decisions may be more related to hasty or bad judgement rather than to ignorance. So too is it with trust.

Young's account of autonomy allows for situations in which a person may not always be in control of their fate and may include some constraints over short-term acts that are not in their long-term interest. These constraints can probably only work if I insist on maintaining certain basic standards and principles and the patient is prepared to trust my judgement on these, although this does not mean I should not explain my position to them. If the doctor–patient relationship is a form of partnership this implies that my integrity has to be honoured as well as the patient's. If I can reasonably explain my strong conviction as the basis for my opinion I should not be coerced into acting against my professional judgment. This is not only a discussion about informed consent, but about the attributes and character of a trustworthy person. It is difficult to override a patient's expressed desires unless the doctor has very clear knowledge of their situation and enduring values. An experienced, empathetic doctor can use their knowledge of how other patients have felt and behaved in similar situations, but it is always difficult to know how a particular patient in a particular situation might feel and react.

In moments of extreme emotion we do not use our rational abilities properly and our decisions may not be authentic until we have had time to calm down and reflect upon them. To be properly self-determining we have to have the capacity to make choices. This includes making choices about our emotions. The patient will decide which emotions are to predominate and which course of action is to be taken. Any action by a doctor, which prevents or diverts the patient from deciding their own course of action, treats the patient as a mere means or a tool, that is, something that is used for another's purpose. Coercion and deception can both do this. Physical coercion treats the patient's physical person as a tool, whereas lying treats their reason as a tool. Because lying interferes with the use of reason it is particularly bad for a Kantian, as it is a direct violation of a patient's autonomy.

Conversely, if a patient's normal rational processes are impaired, it could be considered a duty for a doctor to obstruct the patient in the use of their impaired rational processes, on the grounds that the patient is not exhibiting their true autonomy because they are not able to perform their normal rational thinking. We need to know not only the patient's authentic values and emotions, but also whether their normal rational processes are impaired. To do this it is necessary to distinguish between what is inept judgement and what is impaired by a disease process, trauma, drugs and the like. This is a difficult task but one which doctors face frequently.

Patients also have responsibilities, which include them supplying the doctor with relevant information. Patients sometimes deliberately mislead their doctors for their own gain, for instance by exaggerating symptoms for financial gain in case of litigation or manufacturing symptoms for sympathy and attention. I had a fifty-year-old patient who had had what appeared to be a relatively minor injury to her elbow region at work. She had worked in a factory since leaving school and brought up four children, all the while managing the home and doing all the housework. Her husband did not appear to be much help around the house. I was puzzled why she did not improve. She had persistent swelling in her forearm and hand I could not explain. She remained off work for over a year and ceased doing housework and looking after her children. Her teenage daughters took over the housework and cooking. Her husband still did nothing to help. Whenever she saw me she was usually accompanied by a female relative who fussed over her. Her local doctor and I continued to certify her unfit for work. Eventually she was called to a court to assess her long-term impairment and to determine financial compensation. There was some dispute amongst the medical experts about her elbow movements. The judge asked her to remove a garment covering her arm, a request unusual and unexpected in this setting. To everybody's amazement this revealed she had tied a ligature around her upper arm.

Thus the swelling was explained. She was deliberately causing her arm to be swollen to be relieved of the drudgery in her life and to elicit some sympathy. Unfortunately, she tried for monetary compensation from her employer as well. I confess to feeling some sympathy for her in her family situation but was chastened by the experience. I had trusted her to be open and honest with me.

During my career I was reluctant to operate if I believed a patient did not trust me. One of the most difficult relationships I could have was with a dissatisfied patient, particularly one who was uncertain that they had received the correct treatment and whom I sensed did not trust me. I noticed this tended to occur when I was dealing with a complex problem in which there had been a number of treatment options, for instance in the management of a patient like Robert who had a limb injured by trauma. With severe limb injuries none of the treatment options are likely to give an excellent result and it is not unusual for a patient to face significant long-term disability. It is often the case that a patient has received inadequate information or that he has not fully understood it. Patients can be given misleading advice by friends and other professionals not fully in possession of all the details of the treatment. The combination of misinformation and misunderstanding and poor interpersonal relationships from the medical side can make a patient very angry. Such a patient wants to spend a considerable amount of time discussing their problems and re-establishing some control over their situation. I had to give extra time to these patients and this created problems for me, particularly if I was running a busy clinic and there were many other patients waiting to be seen.

After one such episode I later reflected why I had spent so much time with a patient, when the waiting area was crowded with people, including young children, families and helpers, all people with significant problems often requiring crutches or wheelchairs, thus causing delays for them. These people also deserve my full attention and time. Most doctors do not like having an unhappy patient but I think the major reason I was prepared to give him a lot of time was my belief that he did not trust me. My intuition was that trust is so important and pervasive that it was important not to lose it, even for one person amongst many. I pondered how difficult it would be if every patient in the clinic that morning had questioned me in such detail about the nuances of their treatment. I have no doubt they have every right to do so and when they do question I try very hard to satisfy them. Nevertheless, in the circumstances of my clinic I could not spend all day explaining things. I am not saying that I should not be accountable for everything that I do, nor that patients should not have significant autonomy in decisions made about their treatment, but what does strike me is how much easier it is to work with people in a trusting relationship. As a corollary it is clearly very uncomfortable for a patient to be in a situation in which they do not trust their doctor.

Our relationship had become more complicated than normal: both he and I had had an emotional reaction to each other. He was angry and perhaps inappropriately demanding, I was unprofessionally irritable. Yet at the end of our encounter he was more trusting and I was significantly more satisfied. From then on our relationship went relatively easily.

In this case the patient continued to demand attention beyond what I thought was reasonable and I became irritable and short with him. We both became angry and I walked away to return soon after, a little calmer. Strangely enough, this show of impatience on my part actually seemed to improve our relationship, possibly because we both had time to reflect on what we might lose, and from then on we started to discuss the best way of managing his problem, as though we were meeting together for the first time. At the end of the conversation I asked him whether he trusted me at all. He said he felt he did. Our relationship had become more complicated than normal: both he and I had had an emotional reaction to each other. He was angry and perhaps inappropriately demanding, I was unprofessionally irritable. Yet at the end of our encounter he was more trusting and I was significantly more satisfied. From then on our relationship went relatively easily.

Chapter Seven: Science and Sociology

Trust often appears to be an ephemeral thing. We are aware of its presence but cannot hold it in our hands or define its boundaries. We don't know where it comes from and why it stays or goes. Is there anything tangible and measurable that could help us understand it?

Freitag and Traunmuller[50] analysed responses from people in Germany to various questions about trust. As expected they found that people distinguish trust between close friends, family and social structures from a more generalised trust they may have for people, including strangers. As we develop trust in those close to us we are also more inclined to trust others and this extension of particularised trust is encouraged by and developed through positive experiences with strangers and institutions. A positive experience with strangers is essential for developing generalised trust and this can be reinforced by institutions themselves reinforcing trustworthy behaviour and discouraging untrustworthy behaviour and breaches of trust. Representatives of institutions can be important role models and act as examples of how trust can pay off, thus reinforcing generalised trusting and trustworthy behaviour.

Patrick Sturgis[51] and others have investigated a possible genetic basis for trust as 'trusters' are considerably more likely to join political organisations and civic associations, to have confidence in their institutions of government, to have more positive democratic attitudes and to be more tolerant of minority groups. They are also more likely to be optimistic, well educated, financially secure and confident in their own abilities and self-worth. Trust is lowest among divorcees, the unemployed, ethnic minorities with a history of discrimination and those in poor health. At the aggregate level, trust has been shown to be correlated with the total number of associational memberships and indices of democratic governance at regional and national levels. At the country level, aggregate trust is correlated with social similarity across the culture, such as economic development, lower levels of state corruption, income equality and less criminality and juvenile delinquency.

We tend to trust strangers in general, partly because we learn to do this from our experience, beginning with relationships with our parents, the family and then our friends and colleagues, institutions and government. Through learning to cooperate, our inclinations to trust strangers become gradually incorporated into how we normally see the world. Flanagan and Stout[52] have studied adolescents and measured that their levels of social trust tended to decline through their teenage years and then consolidate as they mature into adults. Their levels of interpersonal trust, however, do not change through these years and students who felt a sense of group solidarity at school and a pride of membership in the institution had a higher sense of social trust than others. Adolescent social trust is shaped by feelings of belonging and collective identity and this corresponds with previous reports that when our human need to belong is satisfied, we all feel better about others. However, strong bonds of trust and loyalty within a group may be at times maintained at the expense of 'outsiders' and 'others'. The students also felt that teachers respecting their opinions and allowing their expression increased their sense of school solidarity, which in turn led to higher social trust. Levels of social trust are higher among adults who, when young, report that their parents and teachers respected their autonomy. Teaching practices that encourage a respectful exchange of views may build feelings of collective identity and solidarity, which, in turn, enhance youth's trust in people. A combination of self-determination and solidarity play an important role in building the stock of social trust that undergirds a democratic society.

Sturgis argues that trust might have a hereditary or genetic element as well as an environmental basis, as there is increasing evidence that interpersonal trust is an important part of personality, with a strong genetically inheritable component. For instance, those people who are generally considered to be 'agreeable' have characteristics that are, at least in part, inherited from their parents. These agreeable people have been shown to have a tendency to trust others, even those who seem to be less agreeable, and thus a tendency to trust might be inherited. In a complex study of twins, Sturgis concludes that trust has a substantial genetic component. Environmental factors also play a major part but he reports that individuals within twin studies are more influenced by particular things that happen to them, that is, their own unique experiences, rather than shared environmental experiences, including all those relating to family and home life. Sturgis does not suggest that parents, for instance, play no role, but rather that in adolescents and young adults individual differences are accounted for by genetics and personal experiences alone. As we get older we tend to become more influenced by the general environment and our experiences with groups and institutions. Studies for genes that may influence social behaviour are potentially unreliable due to their small size, bias in a population study and lack of controls, such as differences within families or between ethnic and cultural groups. Sturgis concedes that all his group may have shown is that trust is an aspect of personality and personality is genetically heritable. Epstein[53], in a study including the heritability of social behavioral phenotypes, suggests that pro-social behaviour is approximately 50% inherited and 50% due to environmental effects, empathy is about 40% hereditary, as is aggression, leadership and parental warmth. In games and tests of trust he estimates the hereditary component is probably of the order of 15%, a small percentage due to the shared environment and about 75% due to the unshared environment, that is, how we have responded to things that have directly affected us. Epstein also concludes that single genes have a very small effect on personality and trust and it is very likely that multiple genes influence these traits.

Paul Zak[54] has examined the Scottish economist and philosopher, and a contemporary of Hume, Adam Smith's work, *The Theory of Moral Sentiments,* and noted that Smith's opinion that 'sympathy' or 'fellow feeling', which we would call 'empathy', that is, a positive emotional response to another's needs, is often rapidly acquired, mostly uncontrolled and strongly emotional rather than cognitive. Zak contrasts this to Smith's more famous book, on economics, *An Inquiry into the Nature and Causes of the Wealth of Nations*, in which Smith postulates that individuals acting in their own self-interest in a competitive environment will produce the greatest overall wealth. Zak also notes that people can be 'rationally rational', that is, they will invest scarce cognitive resources in solving a problem only when the expected payoff is sufficiently large, otherwise they will accept 'good enough'. The brain has evolved to preserve scarce resources and energy and tends to prefer to use learned behaviour in most circumstances, rather like some types of trust.

Daniel Kahneman[55] describes our brains as working as in two systems. System One runs subconsciously and allows us to react automatically and quickly with little or no effort. It has probably developed through our evolution to allow us to recognise and act immediately to dangerous situations. System One may also help us recognise those people who may be a threat and those whom we can probably trust. It allows us to recognise various friendly and unfriendly facial patterns and expressions, detect hostility in a voice, move suddenly when startled and react fearfully to a snake or spider, all before we are consciously aware of these things. Some of these functions we appear to be born with, such as a fear of spiders, and others we learn over a period of time, such as the reading and understanding of social situations. System Two is akin to the way we think of ourselves and involves conscious effort. We can further examine whatever startles us then consider the evidence and decide whether to trust someone. System Two allows us to formulate and solve problems, check the validity of a complex logical argument and engage in abstract thought. System Two has some ability to change the way System One works and instruct us to look for and pay attention to particular features or problems before they happen. Both systems are active when we are awake with System One continually bringing up impressions, intuitions and feelings for System Two to evaluate. System Two is intrinsically lazy and whilst one of its functions is to sometimes overrule the impulses of System One, it often leaves it to go along with 'whatever feels right at the time'. One other thing System One does, in connivance with System Two, is take the amalgam of sensory input it receives and convert it into the simplest and reasonably plausible scenario it can imagine. Thus it is, and we are, sometimes very bad at the type of thinking required for good decisions and we may jump wildly to all sorts of irrational decisions and biases. Spontaneous decisions to trust may share the same characteristics. Of course the two systems are a fiction, or merely an oversimplified way of understanding a complex problem and how to think about judgment and choice.

The human hormone oxytocin has been shown to enhance bonding and care between parent and child, and partners in monogamous relationships. A closely related hormone, arginine vasopressin, also facilitates attachments to mates. At the same time, two other hormones, dopamine and serotonin, each stimulated by oxytocin, can improve social relationships. Simply put, dopamine motivates us to seek rewards such as food and sex and reinforces this by making us feel good about it. Serotonin produces a positive mood and reduces anxiety. Working together, these hormones may help us connect to and behave well towards others and make social reactions pleasant. After an initial positive reaction, if we become increasingly stressed we are increasingly less likely to listen to and be empathetic to each other.

Oxytocin[56] was the first hormone identified: by Henry Dale in 1909. Dale noticed that extracts of pituitary gland caused uterine contractions and the name oxytocin comes from the Greek for 'quick birth'. The hormone was later shown to be important for breast milk production and secretion. Oxytocin also makes mammals calmer, less anxious and more attentive to their babies. As well as dopamine and serotonin, oxytocin acts with the chemicals nor-adrenaline, oestrogen and testosterone, the so-called 'molecules of emotion'. Moderate stress and the subsequent release of moderate amounts of adrenaline and cortisol increases oxytocin levels, whereas high stress and high levels of adrenaline and cortisol reduces oxytocin levels. Oxytocin is manufactured in the hypothalamus and may be secreted directly from there or stored in and secreted from the pituitary gland. The hypothalamus, pituitary and adrenal glands, which secrete adrenaline and cortisol, form a coordinated hormonal axis. This axis is complimented by the sympathetic and parasympathetic nervous systems, which have a wide range of complementary automatic controlling functions. The limbic system of nerves at the base of the brain adjacent to the hypothalamus acts as a centre that processes external stimuli, such as threatening behaviour, and initiates an immediate subconscious reaction to that, such as the familiar fight or flight response that may lead to action without conscious cerebral involvement. The amygdala is at the front of the limbic system and stimulates an emotional reaction, such as fear, to the external stimulus, which may be modified by the hormonal axis in response to signals from other areas, depending on past learnt experience. In certain circumstances oxytocin may calm our fears and in others noradrenaline may enhance them. For instance, a study has shown that men who are shown images of threatening or fearful faces are calmed by the prior ingestion of oxytocin.

The body cells may or may not have receptors for oxytocin, which bind and utilise the hormone, and the cell does not respond without them. A receptor is a chemical that bonds with a hormone that allows the hormone to express itself in that cell. The oxytocin receptors are scattered throughout the body, for instance in the uterus, breast and various parts of the brain, and the number and distribution of the receptors varies considerably between individuals. In the brain they are usually found in large numbers in areas handling interpersonal relations. Oxytocin does not act on a cell unless it binds with a receptor in that cell. Kogana and others[57] describe the oxytocin receptor as a key to social activity, particularly empathy. With oxytocin only some cells express the effects of the hormone and these effects depend on the function of the cell. In the muscle cells of the uterus oxytocin enhances contraction and in the breast it facilitates lactation. In brain cells it may have multiple effects, some of which are related to social behaviour. Oxytocin has just one type of receptor so that any variation in the gene that codes the receptor to carry out oxytocin signaling may influence different social behaviours.

Oxytocin secretion is normally stimulated by activities such as touching, hugging and sexual activity, and levels in the blood and brain may be raised in both the recipient and giver. Even activities such as stroking a dog will raise the level in a human and there is some evidence also in the receiving dog. Oxytocin receptors are present in the brain in relatively small numbers at birth and increase in number over the first three years of development. Their presence appears to be stimulated by mothering and develop in areas that handle social interaction. When a crying baby is picked up by its mother and comforted, oxytocin levels are increased in both. The baby is stressed by things such as being left alone, pain or having a soiled nappy, and the amygdala at the base of the brain generates a fear response. When the mother comforts her the secretion of oxytocin stimulates the production of dopamine, which makes the baby calm. With repeated episodes the habit is learnt and over these early years patterns are established and the baby develops an enduring feeling of comfort and safety, which may contribute to the development of trust. Later in life the response may be triggered by memories, such as of her mother's voice or other kind voices or facial expressions, even from a stranger. The absence of positive caring responses from a mother or other carers may lead to a lack of oxytocin and depletion of the receptors, which in turn may lead to feelings of abandonment, fear, anger and lack of trust that may continue into adult life.

Increasing oxytocin levels increases eye contact and facial recognition between individuals and improves our ability to infer the emotions and intentions of others by observing their facial expressions. Oxytocin does not just improve our attitude towards others, it helps us connect with and understand them. Moreover, the moderate distress of others increases our empathy towards them and our subsequent desire to help them, whereas if we observe a high degree of stress in others we are inclined to withdraw from them. Zak has measured an association between empathy and the brain's release of oxytocin and has shown that if a person trusts a stranger the recipient's oxytocin levels also rise. With increasing oxytocin levels both truster and trustee become more trusting and trustworthy.

Zak concludes that oxytocin appears to subtly alter the balance between the appropriate levels of trust and distrust of strangers, moving people towards greater trust. In his studies an increase in oxytocin significantly increases generosity and empathy and he claims this adds support to Adam Smith's view that fellow feeling motivates us towards virtuous actions. Zak takes a greater and more contentious leap that the 'tiny and ancient molecule' oxytocin, and the neurotransmitters it modulates, appear to be responsible for moral sentiments. More likely, it plays an important, and perhaps essential, part in a complex interaction of a number of factors. Oxytocin and vasopressin have both been associated with long-term pair bonding between animals. Zak has also noted an association between a small group of individuals whose oxytocin levels do not rise after a trust stimulus and who do not subsequently reciprocate trust and he postulates that this group is also inclined to deceive others and have difficulty forming friendships and romantic attachments.

In one study observers were able to tell a stranger's genetic disposition to empathy by watching a short silent video recording of the person listening to their partner discussing a distressing problem. Observers were able to recognise specific non-verbal sympathetic responses and those people who showed such responses were more likely to have a particular genetic variation to the oxytocin receptor that related to pro-social behaviour and the ability to read other people's emotions in reaction to stress. The oxytocin receptor has various forms, or polymorphisms, and we do not have a specific empathy or caring gene. We inherit different copies or alternative forms of genes, called alleles, and the genetic variation associated with oxytocin receptors inherited from our parents can be called the A allele or the G allele. We can inherit AA, AG or GG. There is evidence that the G allele, which evolved first in our evolutionary development, tends to makes us more sociable and the A allele, which came later, tends to make us less social and less empathetic. How these alleles are expressed, or manifested in our reactions and behaviour, depends on the other genetic makeup of an individual and their environment. The studies show that observers looking at other people could, in a very short time, tell whether they had a strong G allele, just by the way they were acting. This suggests that we are really good at picking up on first impressions. Similarly, how we subsequently react can be expressed outwardly by us so that strangers can pick it up. The GG genotypes tend to react in a more caring way whereas AA and AG types have self-reported lower levels of positive emotions, such as empathy and parental sensitivity and perhaps have a higher risk of conditions like autism.

The facial clues to cooperation and trust are complex. Stirrat and Perrit[58] noted that when observing the faces of others for emotion, we tend to concentrate on their transient expressions, however, there are some stable facial features linked to behavioral tendencies. The relative width of the face compared to its vertical length is in part related to hormonal balances in adolescence and a relative increase in facial width is associated with higher adolescent testosterone levels, which in turn has been linked to dominant behavior and reactive aggression. Stirrat and Perrit showed a group of students a picture of a person against whom they were playing an experimental trust game. They had no other information about this person. They concluded that male participants with higher facial width ratios were more likely to exploit their counterparts' trust than the male participants with lower facial width ratios. This did not apply to women, who trusted less and reciprocated positively less on average than the males. Men with wider faces behaved in a less trustworthy manner and were also trusted less. That is, they were intuitively treated as less trustworthy. When showed paired photographs of individuals, where these photos had been digitally adjusted so that in one the person appeared to be long faced and in the other wide faced, participants were significantly more likely to choose images with the lower facial width ratio as being more trustworthy.

Another study led by Seltzer[59] showed that seven- to twelve-year-old girls were comforted following a stressful episode by being held in their mother's arms, but their oxytocin levels rose just as much if their mothers spoke to them on the phone. The girls were comforted by any positive response from their mothers. Seltzer speculates that women in particular, perhaps because of their vulnerability, have developed the ability to use social bonds 'to tend and befriend' and to diminish stress either by seeing, touching or talking. Trust allows couples to be vulnerable with each other and can deepen love and friendship. In a study of women given random electric shocks to the feet, Gottman[60] showed that their anxiety and distress was associated with increased activity in the limbic system, the site of flight and fight responses. If a happily married woman held hands with her loving, trusted husband she was calm and the limbic system was shut down. If she was less happily married there was less affect and holding hands with a stranger produced no affect. Similar good results were achieved after an oxytocin nasal infusion. In games such as the Prisoners Dilemma high trusters are trustful when there is no reason to be suspicious and they are not more gullible than low trusters. Fehr discusses 'betrayal aversion' where we avoid trusting if we believe there is an increased chance of being cheated, which is different to risk aversion. We have a special aversion to being a sucker or being exploited by an untrustworthy partner, independently of our assessment of the actual numerical or practical risks in a transaction.

In 1992 Di Pellegrino and others[61] placed electrodes into neurons in the brains of monkeys that responded when the monkeys picked up a piece of food. They noticed some of these neurons also responded when the monkeys saw a person pick up a piece of food. Later papers showed similar responses to mouth actions and facial gestures. These neurons were subsequently called 'mirror neurons'. Since then, imaging of human brains has shown areas that respond similarly to doing and observing various actions. It has been suggested and enthusiastically accepted by many that mirror neurons mediate an understanding of the actions of other animals and thus the development of empathy. There have, however, been a number of studies casting doubt on these conclusions although it remains a promising area for further research.

Trusting relations are based on a complex interaction between many genetic, developmental, social, emotional, neurological and psychological factors. They depend on both rational and irrational expectations and are bolstered by complex hormonal and neurological interactions probably underpinned by a process of natural selection.

Chapter Eight: Medical Betrayals

In seventy years I may have perpetrated many acts of betrayal, some profound, most less so. Some I am aware of, many I am not. The books I read, plays I see and the films I attend are often centered on acts of betrayal, perceived and real, all of various degrees of importance to the participants and, indeed, to those who may observe the activities. Some people may seem to be unduly sensitive to and upset by a betrayal when a dispassionate observer may not see much of a problem and in other situations an outsider may see a betrayal where the participants do not.

I have shown some examples where it is difficult for patients to understand and comprehend information and also where it is difficult for a doctor, for various reasons, to communicate it. This has assumed that any misunderstanding was due to poor communication and not deceit. One of the attributes of a trusting relationship must be that the truster has some faith that the trustee, to the best of their knowledge and ability, is giving them information that the trustee genuinely believes to be as correct as possible. To trust somebody involves some expectation that they will behave in a certain way and if we suspect or discover that they are misleading us the expectation loses its meaning. One of the problems of self-regulation is that a profession may not keep in touch with public opinion, discount the views of outsiders and forget the importance of the trust the community needs to have in them. Here is an example of a doctor–patient relationship in which a patient was deceived and in which a regulatory body, which is meant to protect the community, may have failed to realise the importance of trust. I contend the regulatory body failed to fully alert the profession to its own interest as well as that of patients.

The Medical Practitioner's Board of Victoria provides an Annual

Report to the Victorian Parliament. The 1995 report of the Board states that 'the prime purpose of medical registration remains the protection of the public'.[62] The Board provides summaries of some examples of matters investigated by them through an informal hearing process. These are a guide 'as to what constitutes unprofessional conduct of the less serious category'. I quote from one such summary:

> Dr J. appeared before an Informal Hearing Panel following a complaint that he had deceived a patient. This patient had engaged in unprotected sexual intercourse on the night before consulting Dr J. She requested he prescribe the 'morning-after pill' to reduce the chances of her becoming pregnant. Dr J. established that the patient had just finished her period and advised her she would not be fertile at that time. The patient nevertheless insisted on the treatment and her demand was unaffected by a description of the possible side effects. Dr J. gave her four placebo tablets instead of the active medication.

> Subsequently the patient discovered this deception and complained to the Board. At the Informal Hearing Dr J. explained his action in terms of 'saving the patient from side effects'. He stated he had never heard of pregnancy occurring at this part of the cycle. The Panel acknowledged that conception in this situation was extremely unlikely but admonished Dr J. for deceiving the patient. Dr J. was advised that he should have either prescribed the tablet sought or given no prescription. Dr J. was reprimanded for conduct which the Panel regarded as unprofessional, 'but not of a serious nature'.

An examination of the Board's decision vindicates their conduct in admonishing Dr J. The patient was given a description of the possible side effects of the treatment that she was able to balance against her fear of pregnancy. No matter how unlikely Dr J. considered pregnancy was, the patient was capable of making a reasonable informed choice.

I would like to leave aside any argument that Dr J's personal moral integrity, perhaps constituted by a belief that the 'morning-after pill' is a form of abortion, might justify his behaviour. He could easily have told her of any underlying moral agenda he may have had. Nor will I discuss any paternalistic argument, such as that Dr J. judged he was acting in the patient's best interest, or any other argument that might condone his behaviour. Whilst I agree with the Board's decision that Dr J.'s conduct was inappropriate, it is possible there are others who may not and I choose not to discuss this. My point of contention is not that the Board was wrong, as I believe they were not, but with their view of Dr J's action being 'not of a serious nature'. Dr J. deceived his patient. I do not know the patient but I imagine she must have felt betrayed. I will argue that this betrayal was a deep wrong, the serious nature of which was underestimated by the Board. There is a distinction between what is merely wrong or mistaken and what is intentionally deceitful. Deception is making others believe what we ourselves do not believe.[63] Dr J. deceived his patient by making her falsely believe that the drug he prescribed her was the one she sought.

Telling the truth may not always seem to us to be the right thing to do. It may be wrong to destroy someone's false beliefs if this leaves them feeling hopeless and alone. One can injure people by destroying their privacy with gossip and we can be cruel to people by not having respect for their feelings. A lie may also be an appropriate defence of privacy when someone is too intrusive. Yet we all know that when we are lied to it is usually to our disadvantage and when we are deceived we feel wronged. We may have no way of distinguishing between true and false statements and if we find one statement is false, we may assume that all are false. It is very easy to lose trust in these circumstances. If doctors persistently deceive patients, even with good intentions in order to reassure them, they will eventually not be believed even when they do tell the truth.

Liars work well in a trusting environment and the more people trust the more vulnerable they are to lies. Kant[64] insisted on an unconditional duty of truthfulness, claiming that a lie always harms mankind generally, even if it appears sometimes to do individual good. Even though most of us can think of examples when we consider it right to lie, liars tend to place a more benevolent interpretation upon their deceits than those who are deceived. Whilst some may argue that deceit is always harmful, and others that deceit is usually harmful but in some circumstances can be justified, society cannot function well without a general respect for truthfulness.

Not all deceits necessarily lead to what we would call betrayal. Whilst I postulate that Dr J. has betrayed his patient, consider the situation where you are visited at home one afternoon by a religious zealot keen to accept a donation for his cause. If you told the zealot that you had no money in the house, when you did have money, we would consider this a deceit, but not necessarily a wrongful one, as we might not be sympathetic to religious zealots. Furthermore, I doubt if we would consider that you had betrayed the doorknocker. There is something special about Dr J.'s relation with his patient that is different to your relationship with the zealot that gives grounds for the patient to feel betrayed. If we feel Dr J. is a betrayer we are likely to admonish him. If we feel you deceived merely to escape a vexing situation we may admire your ingenuity. Dr J. did not live up to the patient's expectations of what a good doctor ought to do and he betrayed her in two ways. Firstly, she depended on him to give her the medication she needed to make and carry out her own decision and he concealed that he had not done so. Secondly, their relationship depended on his honesty and 'if a relationship depends on honesty and others rely on it, then lying can be an act of betrayal'.[65]

The idea that it is acceptable to lie to patients is still quite strongly held in some areas of the medical profession. It is very easy to give examples of extreme types, such as the common one of a woman fighting for her life after a car accident who asks in a moment of consciousness about her spouse and her three children who have died in the accident. It is a dilemma in this situation, and one might argue that she should not to be told, but this is not clearly in her best interests, from her point of view, as the doctor can have no idea what her real values are, as she may want to know. Dr J. replaced his patient's values with his own. She made her decision based on her own values. The risks of her taking the morning after pill mattered far less to her than the risks of becoming pregnant. Either on Kant's views of accepting the patient as a rational being in herself, or Oakley's arguments for assessing and honouring the patient's enduring values, Dr J. did not act in an acceptable way. The reactions of Mrs Whitaker, who was blinded, and Dr J's patient suggest that neither were prepared to accept the loss of trust simply as a matter of a failure of a rationally based assessment their doctor had made.

There are less emotional, but serious examples of medical deceit, such as a surgeon on the golf course with nine holes to play whose telephone rings to inform them that a patient has an unexpected pain or some post-operative bleeding and they decide the patient's condition cannot be very urgent and completes the game. The patient survives but has had two extra hours of pain and anxiety. Selfishness may be much more mundane than this. The doctor's partner is waiting for a call to tell them when they will be home to be with the children and they are in the bar drinking after the game whilst pretending to be held up attending to a patient.

When I first started to think about betrayal, one of the first things that I thought about was whether I had betrayed patients. My initial reaction was that of course that I had not. This conforms with some evidence that betrayers on the whole do not see themselves in this light. Davison-Crews[66] has described what she calls 'backstabbing' in the workforce, particularly in nursing, and calls this a 'betrayal of someone you trust'. She says such betrayal causes hurt and pain and the betrayed women became bitter, angry and resentful. Tara Roth Madden[67] interviewed more than one thousand women about betrayal and found that ninety-five percent of them said that another woman at the office had undermined them. What is of particular interest is that of these women, not one of them had admitted to having undermined someone else. Madden engages and educates readers with her well-documented belief that women wage an 'uncivil war' against each other in the marketplace. From her interviews with working women at all levels, the author concludes that hopes for a supportive sisterhood are proving vain. Some women stymie themselves, fearing to go 'where the men are' lest they fail and others are inhibited by jealous competitors of their own sex, and men, on their part, occupy 'reserved seating: ringside at the office catfight'.

Davison-Crews comments that:

> The only way that backstabbing will be stopped is if women work together. All women must work towards developing confidence in themselves, extending a hand to help others, taking the risk to be overt, confronting backstabbers and not letting them be role models, communicating with each other the lessons they learn and becoming positive role models. No matter how badly you have been hurt, you need to claim the gift of compassion for yourself and for others. You need to build a strong and supportive network that will not tolerate covert action and that supports and rewards overt behavior. It is an important step to becoming a happy and fulfilled woman in the workplace.

Whilst betrayal may be common in our community, most of us, who all probably have been betrayers at times, do not necessarily recognise ourselves in this role, although sometimes we do when it is too late to do anything about it. When I was a very junior doctor in the year after I graduated, one of my patients was dying and the nurses had asked me to look in on her. The curtains were around her bed and she was very near death. After I had sat with her for a while I heard myself being paged and left her and went to the nurses' station to answer the page. When I was there I noticed that the patient's elderly husband and daughter had arrived. They asked me how she was and I replied 'please wait here and just excuse me for a minute'. I went back to the patient and sat by her for a few minutes until I was sure she was dead. In those days sometimes I was not exactly certain when someone was really dead and I did not want to tell her husband until I was sure she was. I then went and told him she was dead. The first question her husband asked me was 'Did you know she was dying when you asked us to wait outside?' I replied that I had wanted to make sure she was dead before I told them. I immediately saw they were hurt and confused. They were shepherded away by a senior nurse and I doubt if the old man ever saw his wife again. It was years before I realised what the problem had been, as it had not occurred to me that he would have wanted to be with his wife when she died, yet I must have had some intuition about it because I still remember. There had been nothing in my own experience of life that had given me any understanding of how that poor man may have felt and I only gradually came to believe that I had betrayed them by not allowing them their last moments together. Was it a true betrayal? At the time it happened I had not been taught how to manage such a situation and what it must be like to be dying or to be a grieving partner. I had neither the training nor the imagination to manage the situation and could not be trusted as I was not able to understand what was happening. If I was in such a situation now I would have no excuse and hope I have sufficient wisdom to manage such an event with more understanding and compassion.

It seems remarkable how something that can cause so much harm to some can be either not recognised or treated so lightly by those who cause the harm. Betrayal usually seems more important to the truster and on deeper reflection I found that I probably had betrayed patients without thinking of it as a betrayal. Some forms of betrayal that came to mind were not giving patients enough information, hurrying a patient so that I might do something else, not giving full attention, giving away secrets, not being strong enough in opposing the poor actions of other doctors and imposing my values on others.

In my middle years I ran a very busy private practice. The more successful I became the less time I had to see each patient. I would often end the day exhausted and must have made mistakes and missed things and dealt with some patients inadequately. Whilst it is probably true that if you want something done you should ask a busy person to do it, eventually something must give way. To cope with the problems I focused more and more on my work. I vividly remember after spending twenty minutes with a 'new' patient she turned to me and said 'you don't know who I am, do you?' I stopped and looked at her and recognised a woman who I had known quite well for some years and who had stayed with us at a family holiday house not all that long before. I had stopped being aware of patients as real people outside the consulting room. I treated at least some patients with less attention than they deserved. To me this was a professional betrayal although the patients may not always have been aware of it. I have, however, been in situations where I have been too busy because of the overwhelming number of patients coming to a clinic. This was usually due to a shortage of facilities, nurses and doctors, something beyond their control in which the betrayal lies elsewhere.

I classify examples of betrayal in medicine into seven general groups: self-interest, lack of care, lack of respect, failures of understanding, lack of compassion, not maintaining professional skills or acting when impaired. Examples of self-interest that constitute a betrayal can concern financial arrangements, where doctors may own or have an interest in institutions to which they refer patients, or when they recommend procedures that generate a higher fee where a lesser paid procedure would do as well. Surgeons are often paid more to perform operations than to treat a condition non-operatively. Self-interest also appears in ways which are less obvious to patients, for instance, in the interest surgeons take in new techniques, where a major advance like laparoscopic surgery can be practiced widely before the procedure is properly assessed and before the surgeons are adequately trained, or where a new surgical implant is used without adequate trials. Doctors are often interested in trying new treatments and can have pet projects and research activities. It can be very difficult for a doctor to give objective information, including alternative treatments, if they are enthusiastic about a particular project. Self-interest also plays a part in the concept of 'defensive medicine', where doctors order more investigations and sometimes more treatment than is necessary in an effort to reduce the possibility that they might be sued for negligence. Self-interest can also apply to research projects, where patients may not be well informed or where the doctor may have a specific interest in a particular drug, particularly if they are given some incentive and funding by a drug company.

Examples of lack of care for patients can include using poor quality implants and not taking sufficient care with simple methods of cleanliness, such as washing hands between patients. Lack of care can also be manifested in a doctor failing to keep up to date with the latest in their particular field, not maintaining skills, not supervising continuity of care for patients and failing to use procedures that reduce the chances of mishaps, such as clinical guidelines or clinical pathways.

Doctors may treat patients badly by not respecting them and being arrogant. A prime example of this is the inadequate time some doctors spend making sure the patient is properly aware of their condition and not speaking clearly without using jargon. Lack of respect can include not listening, not sharing information and not being honest. Patients can be humiliated by being talked down to or rudely, brushed off, and made to feel insignificant. It makes them feel foolish, affronted, undervalued, demeaned and unjustly treated. Empathy and compassion are cardinal medical virtues that need, in a sense, to be inbuilt, but can be honed and practiced. There is a life-long requirement to avoid acting when impaired by alcohol and other drugs.

All these elements need to be nurtured, supervised and often regulated by the responsible professional bodies. Sometimes it is difficult for the medical colleges to self-regulate as it is hard at times to prove a doctor is impaired, has poor judgment, is unskilled or is acting unprofessionally. Each doctor is entitled to justice and may seek legal protection or sue their peers if they act against them. Legal professionals have appropriately different aims to doctors and tend to act in protecting the rights of individuals rather than the good of society, which they may see is a matter for government. It is difficult to get a suitable balance

Other examples of betrayal are not so easy to categorise. The example of the man with HIV/AIDS, frequently given in ethical texts, where a doctor tells the patient's previously ignorant partner of the diagnosis, would probably be seen by the patient as a betrayal. Yet it is a betrayal that may be justified by the community, the partner and the doctor involved. Whilst many would condemn the patient for not telling their partner of the diagnosis, the patient has trusted the doctor with this knowledge and their sense of betrayal may be no less in spite of general opinion that their actions are selfish and destructive. The doctor has to make a choice about who or what they are to betray: their public health role, the patient or the partner. I can also think of situations where I might have betrayed a patient for good reasons, in the sense that I may have been concerned about a sick child at home or another patient who was even more ill. My idea of being a betrayer might therefore vary, depending on the circumstances, as my idea of being a good doctor and acting in expected ways might depend on the circumstances. Nevertheless, I have betrayed patients without being clear in my mind that that was what I was doing.

> ### *I have betrayed patients without being clear in my mind that that was what I was doing.*

Both Dr J's patient and Mrs Whitaker took action against a doctor who betrayed them. Davison-Crews believes that women who have been betrayed should confront the situation, admit that they have been fooled, allow themselves to feel stupid and then confront the backstabber. She says that even if an apology is not forthcoming it is 'a relief to level with somebody'. She believes that expressing feelings and emotions in one way allows the betrayed to get on with their lives. Another way to confront the situation is to take legal action, as Mrs Whitaker did. It is an unfortunate side effect of modern living that doctors are often advised by their legal advisers never to admit liability, although we are now encouraged to express sympathy and regret that something has gone wrong. This may be a safe practice from a legal point of view, but it didn't help Mrs Whitaker resolve her hurt through open discussion. To do this she probably had to take recourse to the law, as she may have been unable to assert herself in any other way.

The following case illustrates another response to a betrayal and suggests that having more-than-average power and knowledge is still no guarantee against it. In 1991, a friend, colleague and fellow student, Dr Charles Eccles-Smith, a General Practitioner in his sixties and a man with considerable experience, underwent coronary artery bypass surgery because of coronary artery disease that was causing him chest pain and a limited ability to exercise. Following the operation he noticed he was no longer able to think as clearly as he had prior to the surgery and he gave up the Master's Degree course we were doing. It was not until after the surgery that he noticed a decrease in his cognitive abilities and discovered that this was a common complication of the procedure, which had been documented, amongst other places, in the widely read British journal, *The Lancet*. Charles had not read these articles, as no doctor has the time to read everything that is published, but he expected his surgeon would have known and advised him of it. Charles and Justin Oakley researched the information that was available to patients in written form from six Victorian Hospitals that performed this type of surgery. Charles did not interview all the surgeons, so he was not aware of what information they gave to their patients, but he was able to remember that his surgeon had not given him any information of this sort. Four of the hospitals had presented information to patients on the neuro-psychological risks prior to surgery, but these risks were described as minor and patients were told to expect recovery in several weeks. However, the medical literature had suggested that more than one third of coronary artery bypass patients continued to experience neuro-psychological problems for more than a year after surgery. Two hospitals supplied this information in a post-operative booklet, too late for any reasonably informed consent to have been made by the patient. Charles claimed that if this information had been available to him prior to his surgery he might not have made the decision to have it, or at least have delayed the surgery until he had finished his thesis. Charles published an article with Justin Oakley criticising the lack of information and recommending ways in which the situation could be improved.[68] In their article they claim that a basic ingredient of a good doctor–patient relationship is the practitioner's respect for the patient's autonomy and that the consent procedures in place in Victoria for this type of surgery were inadequate to protect this autonomy. They recommended that medical practitioners should make core disclosures, which are usually considered material for a particular procedure, to all patients, but also include any extra matter that is material to a particular patient. 'Judging what is material to a particular patient requires being open to the possibility that the patient may have plans, values, and activities quite different from those which the practitioner has or expects others to have.' The general thrust of the conclusions from the article is remarkably similar to that of the High Court decision reached independently, also in

1992, in *Rogers* v. *Whitaker*.

The pamphlets published by the hospitals would have been produced with some care and thought, yet they left out fundamentally important information. It is likely that the information on the possible effect on cognition was deliberately left out, either because it was regarded as not important or in order not to discourage patients from having this 'beneficial' procedure. If the surgeon and the people who produced the pamphlets were challenged, and it was suggested that they had betrayed Charles, then it is likely that they would be shocked at the idea that they were betrayers and would strongly deny it. This betrayal resulted from their failure to think through the ramifications of the effect that the lack of information could have on their patients as it removed the patient's fundamental right to have some say in what happens to his body.[69] The failure appears to be one in which a profession, through its members, perhaps thinking it should appear to act in the patient's best interest, was acting its own interest, as it misled the patient in order to encourage them to have an operation. This is not to suggest that the profession deliberately went out of its way to betray Charles, but that it was a betrayal nevertheless, was not inadvertent and was related to the structure and ethos of the profession. Subsequently the hospitals modified their pamphlets. This is not an isolated incident. Soon after this I wrote a paper[70] giving an example in which a pamphlet published by radiologists misled the public by downgrading the significant risk of a spinal investigation. The pamphlet was changed by the radiologists when they were made aware of it.

What is considered a betrayal will often depend on a combination of circumstances and perceptions. There is one situation where there is general agreement about an absolute betrayal and where a doctor should know that they are betraying his patient. For many centuries there have been reports of sexual relationships between physicians and patients. The Hippocratic Oath forbids it.[71] In spite of this, Kerdner[72] discovered up to ten percent of doctors admit to having engaged in erotic behaviour of some sort with patients. Doctors who claim that sexual relationships with patients are sometimes acceptable may attempt to justify their activities if they believe that there is a genuine feeling in the relationship. They may also claim that they are acting as some form of parental surrogate for the patient, thus assisting the 'child' that they argue exists in every adult patient. Kerdner discusses the parallels between sexual activity between doctors and patients and that of childhood sexual exploitation and claims that the doctor who abandons their role as a carer to become a lover effectively 'orphans' their patient and leaves them more vulnerable than when they entered the relationship. Luepker[73] noted the parallel between physician sexual misconduct and child sexual abuse and agrees that, as most patients place a special trust in their doctor, sexual misconduct violates that trust in the same way that it violates a child's trust in an adult abuser. In some instances the patient initiates the sexual relationships and thus it may appear that the patient has made their own choice, but the psychiatric literature suggests this is likely ultimately to be to their disadvantage. It also illustrates the complexities of a trusting relationship where the trustee may have something to gain and does not acknowledge or control this.

The doctor who initiates sexual activity with a patient knows that this is unacceptable yet does it for his own gratification. This gratification may stem from some need to have power, increase their self-esteem or perhaps some need to be loved or even controlled by others. The therapists of sexually abused patients have occasionally observed parallel role reversals. Hyams[74] states:

> Among the most striking role reversals are those when a parent or therapist begins to rely on the child or client for emotional support and guidance. The parent who shares his marital troubles with the child and asks to be taken care of bears a stark similarity to the therapist who spends the client's session talking about his or her personal problems and then asks the client to fulfil unmet needs'.

Kerdner adds:

> The physician's protestation that by being his patient's lover he is really proving he cares and is therefore offering

a valuable gift, is best viewed as an emotional Trojan horse that conceals not only his own needs, but hostility and antipathy towards his patients as persons and their struggle for emotional wellbeing.

A doctor who has these needs does not have the virtues required to be in this position of trust and their choice of vocation needs to change away from patient contact. A profession that does not insist on this risks losing the general trust of the community.[75] Potential betrayers could be alerted by the medical profession defining betrayal and its effects as clearly as possible. This may encourage them to think more clearly about the consequences of their actions.

A patient needs to know certain facts about the doctor. These include their skill, competence and reliability, external interests that might interfere with their care and any physical, psychological or social factors that may impair their ability to carry out any necessary decisions and tasks. It is also important to know the sort of person the physician is and whether they have the attributes necessary to be trustworthy. Unfortunately, none of this information allows a patient to discern the physician's 'practical wisdom', something which may be a very important part of the relationship. There are ways to assess the medical competence of a doctor, although these methods are at present inadequately applied and rarely made available for general publication. Initially a patient could rely on the doctor's general standing in the community and their reputation as a good doctor. This may seem a reasonable general guide, but we all know that those who publicise themselves or advertise their skills are not necessarily the best doctors, although they may well be competent entrepreneurs. Governments, insurers and hospitals are increasingly requesting that surgeons supply outcome data to assess their performance. It is possible to monitor factors like post-operative complications and infection rates for individual surgeons and to demand evidence of continuing education and the updating of skills.[76] Some have suggested the use of 'report cards' on individual surgeons and hospitals and this is an attractive idea, although it may be difficult to obtain meaningful data. Often the most experienced surgeons treat the most difficult problems and their results may not look as good as those doing easier work. Poor performance can be assessed but the information is often not collected, made available or acted upon.

To be considered worthy of trust in an increasingly complex society surgeons will have to be much more open about their own performance, take a greater interest in the performance of their colleagues and be prepared to publicise their results. There will be some difficulties if a hospital releases statistics of their results and complication rates, and grades them from the surgeon getting the best results and the least complications down to the surgeon getting the worst results and the most complications. There may be logistical problems if this is done, as if it becomes clear that one doctor is the best surgeon, then one would assume that the vast majority of patients would wish to see them and might be disappointed if they were not able to do so. Most patients would be unhappy if somebody they considered fourth best was treating them. Having established, if it were possible, who the best cardiac surgeon was, they would not be able to cope with all the work that they would have to do once everybody demanded their services. This does happen to an extent in developed countries and it is the financially well off who seek those surgeons out. To overcome these problems we have to aim for a general level of acceptable, verifiable, minimum standards. The actual maintenance of standards, once established, may have to be left to the profession, as only a doctor can assess the skills of another. This implies a much more rigorous application of professional standards and some sort of independent external supervision. This is not to say that the community cannot also insist on having doctors who possess virtues, such as empathy, compassion and veracity, which all can recognise. Fortunately, whilst there are surgeons who are exceptionally good and some who are exceptionally bad, the vast majority, as far as I can tell, are reasonably competent.

As doctors get older they may have impaired memory and cognitive skills and may not necessarily be aware that their performance is decreasing or, if they are, may deny it. There is a significant incidence of alcoholism and drug abuse amongst doctors that may impair their judgement and performance. It is also possible that a surgeon could be HIV positive or have other infectious diseases that he might pass onto a patient. There has been a recent case in Australia where an anaesthetist was found guilty of infecting a number of patients by injecting himself with some of the anaesthetic agents before using the same needle to inject them into a patient. There are organisations available to advise doctors damaged by drugs or illness and these depend on the voluntary cooperation of the members. This is a difficult area, as whilst the profession is interested in protecting itself from outside scrutiny, there are also genuine concerns about the just management of the ill or impaired doctor.

In an attempt to protect patients from poorly performing or dangerous doctors legislation has been introduced in Australia to force mandatory reporting of doctors in certain circumstances. A reporting practitioner or employer must have formed a reasonable belief that another practitioner:

> 1. Practiced the practitioner's profession whilst intoxicated by alcohol or drugs; or

> 2. Engaged in sexual misconduct in connection with the practitioner's profession; or

> 3. Placed the public at risk of substantial harm in the practitioner's practice of the profession; or

> 4. Placed the public at risk of harm because the practitioner has practiced the profession in such a way that constitutes a significant departure from accepted professional standards.

There have been concerns that this might stop unwell doctors from seeking help, but an unwell practitioner whose health has been well managed and the public is not at risk does not require reporting. There are various health plans available for doctors who are unwell although sick doctors do not always recognise they need help or seek it. In general, mandatory reporting raises concerns about serious issues and less obvious issues are not so clear cut.

Manson and O'Neill would like to see robust and transparent systems of accountability established to enhance the trustworthiness of doctors. They claim good systems of accountability do increase trustworthiness, but those who rely on these systems are in effect placing reliability on 'second order systems' where primary workers show to others whether or not they are performing well and are held accountable for this. The managers who supervise the primary workers do not necessarily understand the work being done and often set up convenient and uniform measures, which appeal to the managers, but in effect do no more than appear to hold others to account. This undermines the primary workers and their 'professionally informed judgment' as meaningful outcomes are very hard to measure, particularly complex problems requiring judgment, which, as we have seen, is often a matter of perception. Yet, as we have also seen, professionals may be too close to other professionals to rigorously hold them to account, so whilst their judgments are informed, they are not independent. Transparency may be helpful but it is easy to fudge results and they are limited by questions of confidentiality and problems with interpretation and understanding. Somewhere there has to be an open, combined, form of judgment. Thus far there is no evidence that increasingly sophisticated methods of accountability have shown any difference in the level of the public's trust of doctors and nurses, which mostly remains high.

Chapter Nine: Institutions

Charles Cullen started killing patients in hospitals in the eastern part of the United States in 1988. Working as a nurse it is estimated he possibly killed over 300 in the next 15 years and he confessed to killing up to 40. He moved from hospital to hospital, often after suspicion of his conduct was raised by his fellow staff members. He was first suspected by hospital authorities soon after the killing began, after an investigation of contaminated intravenous bags concluded that he was most likely responsible for some deaths. Nothing further was done except he was asked to leave and he continued to find work in other hospitals, often because there was a shortage of nurses. During this time he had treatment for multiple suicide attempts and mental illness yet there was no mechanism available to recognise nurses with mental health and employment problems. In 2002 in yet another hospital, authorities were notified by his co-workers of their suspicions, but the fears were dismissed because of an alleged lack of evidence. Later it was found that the hospital had obstructed the investigation by withholding evidence. Eventually, in July 2003, a poisons centre advised a hospital of various suspicious drug overdoses. Perhaps to avoid further investigation, Cullen was dismissed for lying in his job application. He was arrested in December 2003, after more patients had been killed. Cullen was not alone in perpetrating similar crimes. Orville Majors, a nurse in Indiana, was convicted of killing a number of patients between 1993 and 1995. He may have killed up to 130 and was discovered when it was noted that the patient mortality rate doubled when he was on duty and the hospital's overall mortality had tripled since he had been employed.

The reasons given for the failure to apprehend Cullen include the lack of a requirement to report suspicious workers, minor penalties for failing to report, inadequate legal protection of employers, no authority for employers to investigate employment and fears of lawsuits for giving a bad reference. Since 2003 many legal changes have been made in the USA, including New Jersey where licensed healthcare professionals have to undergo criminal background checks and be fingerprinted.

Yorker[77] and her colleagues investigated 90 criminal prosecutions of healthcare providers for the serial murder of patients between 1970 and 2006 in twenty countries, forty percent of which were in the United States. Fifty-four of the 90 have been convicted, 45 for serial murder, four for attempted murder and five pleaded guilty to lesser charges. Following the investigation a further twenty-five have been indicted and are either waiting trial or the outcome has not been published. Injection was the main method used by the killers, followed by suffocation, poisoning and tampering with equipment. Nursing personnel comprised 86 percent of those prosecuted, physicians 12 percent, and allied health professionals two percent. The number of patient deaths that resulted in a murder conviction was 317 and the number of suspected deaths was 2013. The authors concluded that these numbers are disturbing and demand the implementation of systemic changes in tracking adverse patient incidents associated with the presence of a specific healthcare provider. They suggest that hiring practices must shift away from preventing wrongful discharge or denial of employment lawsuits to protecting patients from employees who kill.

In January 2000 a British General Practitioner, Dr Harold Shipman, was found guilty of murdering 15 of his patients and has been suspected of deliberately killing about 250 between 1975 and 1998, most, but not all, being elderly women. He had a pattern of giving his victims lethal doses of diamorphine, signing their death certificates and then falsifying their medical records. In early 1998 Deborah Massey, of Frank Massey and Sons Funeral Parlour, prompted a fellow partner in Shipman's practice to approach the police about the large number of cremation certificates that Shipman was having countersigned. Death certificates can be signed by a doctor who knows of a patient's condition at the time of her death, but a cremation certificate needs to be countersigned by a non-treating doctor who has to be satisfied there is no reason to suspect why she should not be cremated. The police found insufficient evidence to take any action.

In June 1998 another patient, Kathleen Grundy, died in Shipman's care and this time her daughter went to the police, as Kathleen had recently changed her will in favour of Shipman. Her body was exhumed, as she had not been cremated, and was found to contain diamorphine. Further evidence implicated Shipman and investigation of other deaths linked them to him. Later it was found that Shipman had a history of using illegal drugs and in 1975 had been convicted of forging prescriptions of pethidine for his own use. He had been fined, briefly attended a drug rehabilitation unit and was allowed to continue to practice and he probably continued to use drugs, if only intermittently.

The Shipman Inquiry, established to examine the circumstances of the Shipman case, made many recommendations, including reform of the coroner system, controlled drug prescribing, death and cremation certification, patient complaint systems, appraisal of medical professionals and medical regulation. The enquiry also recommended mortality rate monitoring if it could be shown to be effective in detecting a future mass murderer in general practice. This is difficult to do. At best it can be a backstop to detect a particularly prolific serial killer when other means of detection have failed. Guthrie[78] and others concluded that policy should focus on changes likely to improve detection of individual murders, such as reform of death certification and the coroner system. Of their own volition some doctors in Hyde, the town in greater Manchester where Shipman was in practice, tightened up the part of the cremation certificate that corroborates the cause and circumstances of death stated by the attending doctor. Other doctors introduced systems to allow patients to directly access their own records, partly as a means of restoring the trust of their patients. However, the recommendations of the enquiry faced considerable resistance from many doctors and may have provoked anxiety among them about the risk of increased regulation, monitoring and control. In 2008 Richard Baker[79] commented that:

> But as yet, our profession has not debated the meaning
> for us of the Inquiry's fifth report and how we should
> restore medical professionalism, but instead has focused

most concern on the impact of largely reasonable new government policies. Until the Inquiry's criticism is faced by doctors, it will be impossible to convince policymakers that medical professionalism can be relied on to place patient safety before doctors' interests.

Charles Cullen worked as a nurse in a number of institutions that, in spite of continuing suspicion, allowed him to continue to kill patients. Harold Shipman was a relatively independent doctor, whose activities would have been harder to detect, but could have been stopped much earlier if sufficient attention had been given to the supervision of doctors at risk of offending. A more rigorous approach to the various administrative procedures designed to protect patients and more stringent efforts of his profession in accepting overall responsibility for the behaviour of its members is required.

In June 1998 the professional conduct committee of the General Medical Council of the United Kingdom found three medical practitioners guilty of serious professional misconduct due to the high incidence of mortality in the Bristol paediatric cardiac surgical unit. The central allegations were that two surgeons continued to carry out operations knowing that their mortality rates were unacceptably high. The Chief Executive and the Medical Director of the overriding United Bristol Health Care Trust were aware of the situation and allowed it to continue. Furthermore, the two surgeons were accused of not communicating to the parents the correct risk of death for the operation in their hands. One of the features of the case was not the failure to detect the problem - it was detected – but the fact that the authority took no action on warnings that they had repeatedly received. Even good data is not useful if no one acts on it. A specific problem in Bristol was that one of the cardiac surgeons was also an administrator in the hospital and his colleagues, who were also his friends, were reluctant to take action. As a major advance the Bristol Royal Infirmary decided to publish its comprehensive risk stratified data on its web site. This data was based on recommendations by the Society of Cardiac Surgeons that were then used extensively across the United Kingdom. Since then there has been increasing interest and action in disseminating data about other surgeons and hospitals.[80]

Geoffrey Davies[81], a prominent jurist, asked a meeting of Australian surgeons in 2013 to consider two questions:

> 1. Should you have an effective system for detecting and dealing with your colleagues whose performance is below an acceptable standard?

> 2. Should you make public the death and disability rate of each surgeon in your specialty measured against an expected range based on patient characteristics?

By 'you' he said he meant not as individuals but as a specialist society. He had no doubt that a poll of the general public would yield an unqualified yes, yet pointed out that in Australia, with one exception, surgical societies ignored both questions. Every profession has incompetent members and at various times every professional will be aware of at least one of them. In surgery these people operate in such a sub-standard way that they put patients at risk of injury, disability and perhaps death, yet there is clear statistical evidence that it continues to occur. Davies states that much of this is preventable. One way to do this is to identify those surgeons who err and either retrain them, prevent them from performing operations they do poorly, or in the worst cases stop them practising altogether. Those who participate in surgical audits improve their performance but these are not always compulsory and the identity of particular surgeons is often hidden. One argument for not openly divulging an individual surgeon's results is that it discourages disclosure and frankness, but Davies argues that this suggests surgeons consider self-protection from action against them to be more important than patient safety. The experience in England since 2005 has shown that death rates have dropped since publication began and there is no evidence that surgeons have avoided doing high-risk cases. Davies argues that reporting of patient morbidity should be undertaken openly in a similar way, and makes a compelling argument that a prospective surgery patient has a right to know these rates before choosing a surgeon. At the end of his talk Davies told his audience:

Your presence here today marks each of you as a surgeon who is concerned about the health and safety of patients who come under your care. You should demonstrate that concern by ensuring that your specialist bodies remedy their failure to act. Otherwise are we, the public, to infer from this failure that you are more interested in protecting your incompetent colleagues than you are in the health and safety of surgical patients?

My personal opinion is that underneath we are all afraid of been found out, as we know we make mistakes and fear the possibility that one day we will be found wanting and exposed to public gaze. We also like to support our mates and are reluctant to weaken our professional solidarity. Michael Grigg, the president of the Royal Australasian College of Surgeons in 2015, supports Davies opinion and describes a triangle of trust that must exist between the profession, the public and the state. He believes surgeons have done well in training young surgeons and setting up continuing professional development programmes, but sees the increasing involvement of the state in mandating continuing professional development as an example of the profession's failure to enforce its own standards and to identify and manage those who do not measure up.

There have been many studies over the last decade concerning the high levels of adverse events in hospitals. A good example is in the use of prescribed medicines where serious and sometimes fatal errors can occur. These can include writing in the wrong patient's chart, prescribing the wrong dose, being unaware of known allergies and not recognising drug incompatibilities. This is more common when young doctors are not adequately supervised but can happen quite surprisingly and unexpectedly in the hands of experienced medical specialists. We all sometimes do something quite contrary to our usual practice and can be astounded when we realise what we have done. The airline industry has led the way in analysing these types of events in all of their procedures and safety exercises and has devised lists of the steps to be taken in order. Their emphasis is not on apportioning blame when things go wrong but on rigorous exposure and analysis and the subsequent development of newer, better protocols. My college now runs regular courses with the airline industry to improve our performance in these matters. Of real benefit is the more frequent use of computers in prescribing drugs, as they can easily indicate and warn of a patient's drug history, allergies and incompatibilities. The idea that no one is to blame in most adverse events sits uncomfortably with many, as someone has to be ultimately responsible, but a whole industry or profession taking responsibility for minimising the inevitable well-meant mistakes is encouraging.

The idea that no one is to blame in most adverse events sits uncomfortably with many, as someone has to be ultimately responsible, but a whole industry or profession taking responsibility for minimising the inevitable well-meant mistakes is encouraging.

We often trust government departments and representatives of professions and institutions, such as doctors and nurses in a hospital. Francis Fukuyama defined trust as:

> The expectation that arises within a community of regular, honest, and cooperative behaviour, based on commonly shared norms, on the part of other members of that community.

Fukuyama's definition of trust is based on the implied or publicly expressed attitudes, values and behaviour of others and depends on our knowledge of how our friends, doctors and others have behaved in the past. We believe that certain people ought to behave towards us in certain favourable ways and have obligations towards us.

A patient should reasonably expect his surgeon to perform an operation with due technical competence[82], carefully, soberly and safely. Technical competence can be monitored, not necessarily by the patient but by others, as it is based on shared knowledge and expertise. Surgeons and operating room staff can assess technical competence and a patient placing his trust in a surgeon should be able to expect that these people will also be looking after their interests. Individual surgeons wish to maintain a general level of competence for their own professional benefit if nothing else, and hospital administrators will be concerned, for a variety of reasons, to have and to be seen to have, high standards. Technical competence also implies the application of external standards such as benchmarking. One of the major positive effects of the open publication of the results of cardiac surgery has been the stimulation of competitive health administrators to promote higher standards.

> *One of the major positive effects of the open publication of the results of cardiac surgery has been the stimulation of competitive health administrators to promote higher standards.*

Another public manifestation of trust has to do with expectations of fiduciary obligation and responsibility. Doctors have a responsibility to demonstrate a special concern for the interests of others above their own concerns. They are not always confident that they are as knowledgeable as they or others would like them to be and public expectations may need to be modified in light of their experience and circumstances. Such dilemmas may be partially resolved by doctors acknowledging their limitations, experience and specific expertise. For instance, the results of some complex and uncommon operations, such as surgery on the oesophagus and pancreas, may be better performed in hospitals by teams with special expertise and experience. It is in a patient's best interest to be referred to an experienced team, even if this is socially and financially inconvenient. This requires an open understanding of the location of such centres and the admission of the need to refer patients to them. Included in this requirement is the need for a surgeon to acknowledge his own lack of expertise and for administration to accept this and arrange and support areas of excellence.

One example of the way the law may strengthen this in the future comes from a decision of the High Court of Australia (*Chappel* v. *Hart*, 1998)[83]. Mrs Hart was a lecturer in a tertiary institution and was contemplating surgery for a pharyngeal pouch. A pharyngeal pouch forms due to a weakness in the wall of the pharynx at the upper end of the oesophagus allowing the lining of the pharynx to balloon out. This pouch can fill with food and secretions, and cause difficulty in swallowing. It can also overflow at night and leak into the trachea and lungs, thus causing a cough and infection. Surgical removal of the pouch and repair of the pharyngeal wall is a reasonable and often effective option. Mrs Hart asked about the possibility of her voice changing and becoming husky, as she did not want to sound like a local politician who had this problem. Damage to the recurrent laryngeal nerve, which supplies the muscles controlling the larynx, or voice box, can lead to this and is a well-known complication of operations around the thyroid gland below the pharynx. Dr Chappel, the surgeon, warned of the common risks of his proposed operation but did not include the unlikely possibility of damage to the nerve, as it is not normally at risk in an operation on a pharyngeal pouch. Mrs Hart had some leakage around the operation site and subsequently had inflammation that spread around and below the pharynx and which led to recurrent laryngeal nerve damage. She was successful in her case as the High Court ruled that Dr Chappel should have told her of the risk, remote as it may have seemed to him, as it was material to her. During the proceedings an expert witness testified that he had done the operation frequently without this complication, whereas Dr Chappel had done very few such operations. Mrs Hart therefore claimed she would have gone to a more experienced surgeon if she had known. Although the judgement was based on the question of informed consent, it was the opinion of one of the judges that it should be a doctor's duty to tell a patient if a more experienced surgeon was available. It has been postulated that this opinion may be adopted by a future court.

People want and expect fiduciary responsibilities, not just from individuals, such as doctors, but from institutions, who need to conform to a broad social expectation of their function, that is, to be able to supply technically competent treatment and to fulfil certain obligations and responsibilities. Every patient expects the staff of a hospital, by the nature of its standing in the community, to conform to certain acceptable standards that allows them to trust it. The community itself, having an interest in maintaining a hospital's standards also has a responsibility to preserve those standards.

If we live in relatively small communities we are mostly aware of and understand the people in whom we trust, but in the modern world we often deal with large institutions and have no real idea of what goes on within them. As our experiences of the world grow more complex, so that we are no longer capable of comprehending the whole, trust helps to reduce this complexity in order for us to function.[84] We have little choice but to renounce complete information and control and thus trust becomes a gamble to reduce complexity. Many patients do not make real choices because their decisions often depend on unreliable, deficient or to them, incomprehensible, information. The patient who interrupted me to say she trusted me, may have done so because she was overwhelmed with information, which she may not have fully understood, and simply wanted to reduce the complexity of the situation. In a way this may have reflected a lack of choice on her part and I may have deluded myself that I represented some positive personal factor in our relationship. Her trust might merely have been a device to allow her to cope with her lack of personal control due to our unequal relationship and her incomplete knowledge and understanding, and my failure to appreciate and address this.

Trust as a broad social expectation relies on the persistence of the social order, roughly equivalent to us assuming, for instance, that bridges will last for generations and that human life will survive. These broad social expectations are necessary for everyday life and without some trust of this nature, the world would be so disorganised that we would feel unable to get out of bed in the morning. Within such a broad social expectation, the grounds of trust include expectations of persistence, regularity, order and stability. According to Garfinkel[85], that is 'to be able to take for granted, to take under trust, a vast array of features of the social order'. Garfinkel performed a number of experiments in social disorder, using what he called 'breaching experiments', in which individuals were confronted by abnormal or bizarre behaviour and who reacted by becoming confused, unhappy and aggressive. Our expectations involve some important social constructions that matter to us in the way we live our lives and to which we react unfavourably when they fail.

Reducing complexity depends on an institution having the power to make decisions about individual members of the community without them being aware of either the process of the decision-making or the attitudes of individuals within the institutions. This disenfranchises them from being involved in decisions in any meaningful way. There is a danger, if we are to blindly rely on the internal mechanisms of institutions, that they will be inclined to operate more in their own interests than ours. Ann Daniel acknowledges that the major professions of our time, such as those of law and medicine, have developed a reputation for good work and thus respect and trust. This reputation has become a source of authority for the professions, which 'encompasses the concession of trust implicit in a practitioner's license to practice'. Daniel traces the history of these two professions, showing their dedication to a higher cause and their emphasis on aspects of enacting rituals, adopting specific language and symbols, wearing the robes of their calling and the taking of vows or oaths on entry committing to profess a life of learning and service.

Purtilo and Kassel[86] discuss three criteria that they claim are generally agreed upon as essential characteristics of a profession. Firstly, the members of a profession claim a particular knowledge or competence often associated with specialised education and training. Secondly, they suggest that a profession offers a service that has some significant social value. Thirdly, that a professional usually derives satisfaction from their work because of the service it provides to the client and this satisfaction is added to any remuneration the professional might receive. However, probably the most important aspect of the professions is that they reserve the right to set and evaluate their own standards of quality. They claim this right on the grounds that they are the only ones with the knowledge to properly assess that quality.

Pellegrino and Thomasma[87] claim that we have forgotten the basic ideal of being a professional. They describe how Scribonius Largus used the word 'profession' in the first century AD and how he tied it to a special promise of compassion and aid. They claim that the term 'professional' is now used too widely and has become meaningless. In the medical context they say the term should specify a promise made by the professional to care for the interests of the patient so they can be trusted not to abuse the privileges the promise entails. Their ideal of a health professional includes a commitment that they will not place their own interest before the patient nor will they exploit the vulnerability of a patient. In this way medical professionals, and perhaps teachers, may need to honour different standards than other recognised professionals because of the need for them to make the interests of their patients their primary concern, although this is not to say that lawyers and investment advisors should not also be expected to take note of their client's interests. They go on to argue that health professionals must merit the trust the profession invites and they claim that if they do not rise to those obligations, then they can hardly protest when they are satirised, or treated as a trade or business and regulated as such. The nature of the acts health professionals are expected to perform, together with the trust such acts demand, should form the basis of their professional morality.

The nature of the acts health professionals are expected to perform, together with the trust such acts demand, should form the basis of their professional morality.

Daniel describes a collaboration that exists between the professions and the State, such that a monopoly has been formed to the exclusion of other interests. She contrasts this 'political history' with Foucault's 'critical history' which puts knowledge at the centre of medical authority and influence.[88] Foucault argued the centrality of knowledge, ordered into a specific discourse, legitimates the power of a profession. Daniel also describes a third 'history' of a profession, one presented by sociologists who draw up a catalogue of characteristics apparent in those occupations commonly regarded as professions. She says this catalogue shows what professionals believe about themselves, the knowledge they have and the skills they apply. Knowledge is crucial to professional power and identity and the modern State validates this authority by formally registering the professional bodies. 'Medical Science can be seen as a paradigm case of the ascent of power tied to scientific knowledge and the disciplinary normalisation (standard setting and monitoring) of the learned college'. Daniel believes that such power is difficult to discipline and any discipline that does occur tends to serve the self-interest of the profession and its individual practitioners rather than those they are meant to serve.

There is also always the danger that scientific knowledge, whilst powerful, can be turned to evil as well as good, such as in the experimentation of the Nazi doctors. Daniel believes that the professions should reflect the values of the community. The Nazi doctors represented a very small minority of the profession. The majority of German doctors continued to practice ethically precisely because they did not take the values of the community. Daniel presents a bleak view of the self-centred morality of the medical profession, which, if justified, suggests that individual medical practitioners and their professional body may appear to be trustworthy only to protect their self-interest. Yet the idea that self-interest is often, if not always, the basis of human action is not a new one and it has been challenged before.

As rational thought and knowledge based on personal observation, rather than being imposed by Church and Crown, became widespread in Europe in the sixteenth and seventeenth centuries, the idea that morality could also be based on these concepts was established. Because rationality is the product of individual thought, this led to the gradual evolution of the idea of individual autonomy as the basis for moral values, which in turn led to the concepts of natural rights and social justice. Natural rights originally meant that people could make moral assessments, based on 'natural law', which was God's will on earth. Eventually the term natural law lost many of its religious connotations and natural rights are considered to be those owed to all people, at times almost as though individual autonomy has become 'sacred' in itself.

The seventeenth century English philosopher, John Locke[89] argued that humans were often altruistic. He believed that the contention that humans only act selfishly, 'has always been opposed by those who have a sense of common humanity and concern for the fellowship of man'. He argued that we have always praised altruistic actions and that if the private interest of each person were the only basis of the law, then that law would inevitably be broken, as it is impossible to have 'regard for the interest for all at one and the same time' as sometimes the interests of one must be put ahead of another. The force of Locke's argument lies in his belief that people generally applaud virtuous actions and support the importance of justice and equity:

> What else indeed can human intercourse be than fraud, violence, hatred, robbery, murder, and such like, when every man not only may, but must snatch from another by any and every means that which the other in his turn is obliged to keep safe.

Locke argued that self-interest could never be the basis for a good society as trust was essential for this and if self-interest prevails, 'So all society is abolished and all trust, which is the bond of society.'

Daniel claims, in my view, correctly, that:

> The public presentation and reputation of a profession must go beyond the image of knowledge, expertise and practised excellence and stand for moral concern and responsibility.

The professions must be trustworthy and be seen to be so. Not only is this trustworthiness important for those outside the profession, it is also important for the profession itself, for if trust in the profession diminishes, that profession's reputation and authority also diminishes. Daniel believes the ethics of professions are, in an effort to maintain that profession's integrity and power, invariably directed to the good of the profession and because of this they have increasingly relied on the regulatory powers of the state and the law courts to control any member whose actions threaten them. This reliance on the power of the law has become a double-edged sword for medicine, as the courts may now see themselves as enabled to criticise and control medical practice.

The idea of trust is central to Locke's vision of good government.[90]

Government is a relationship between the people and their leaders, who are capable of deserving trust, but any of whom can and sometimes will betray that trust. Locke believed it was essential that government could be trusted by the people and claimed that men were so aware of this that they were prepared to 'on the whole trust the rulers far beyond the latter's desserts'. Whilst trust is a duty for humans under the law of nature, this did not mean that people should be credulous. The citizens should not take any betrayal by a government or its servants lying down and the remedy for the betrayal of trust was the right of revolution. If a government, or a modern institution, is not trustworthy and is seen to be significantly betraying those it has a duty to protect, then this government or institution ought to be changed. Locke claimed that a person with power over others who betrayed that power was unjustly trying to enforce their own ends and therefore could be justly destroyed. His ideas of justice and equity support the concept that the general public should be aware of and monitor the power of governments, institutions and professions, and take particular care that they are truly trustworthy.

In the broad discussion of trust as a social expectation we have seen that the grounds of this sort of trust are expectations of persistence, regularity, order and stability. We take certain things for granted, such as a regular supply of food, the affection of our families and our social relations. These we have come to accept out of habit and some we appear never to have questioned at all. However, reflection suggests that sometime in the past we have made decisions about many of those things we now take for granted. If, for instance, when driving a car we are confronted with an emergency situation we appear to unthinkingly swerve away, but this activity has not come naturally to us. We have learnt step by step how to use the accelerator, brake and steering wheel, how to judge the distance from the car ahead and various other factors. We practice these activities and make decisions about them until they become apparently effortless, thoughtless, principles of action. Each time we come upon a new situation we make choices and over a period of time build up more principles of action. We use these principles so that we do not have to keep making the same decisions over and over again.

Martha Nussbaum argues that our ethical and social values depend on our upbringing and habits. This means it is not easy to replace them at will as we are 'raised inside' them and 'they are in us'. This gives our values and habits inherent stability but it also continues any inbuilt bias. We do not suddenly trust institutions but develop habits of trusting, often unconsciously, and we can only change these habits if given sufficient reason to do so. As Hegel[91] wrote, 'Faith and trust emerge along with reflection; they presuppose the power of forming ideas and making distinctions.' We could thus make decisions to trust a group or institution by applying principles that we know have served us well in the past.

If you come into any hospital with a serious illness you will soon meet a number of strangers who will make some major decisions about you that are beyond your control. Even though these strangers may be employed by the hospital and are therefore subject to its rules, are members of a profession and accept its ethical and practice standards and acknowledge certain legal duties, they will make decisions about you with a remarkable degree of personal freedom. This freedom they guard jealously and claim they do so to protect your interest. Most of them feel keenly the need to be worthy of your trust. This suggests a corresponding need for you to insist on these strangers being particularly trustworthy. It also means you are very vulnerable to any untrustworthy behaviour. In a world where many people we meet cannot be our friends, a central condition for co-operation and assistance is trust. Whilst families and friends can learn whom they can trust, co-operation between groups and individuals depends on the possibility of trust among people who do not and cannot know each other intimately, but who still must make judgements about the extent to which they can rely on each other. In most hospitals patients may have no opportunity to make any judgements at all.

My relationship with a severely injured patient was a very complex one and included elements of a social contract, legal responsibility, an implied promise for me to act well and a degree of trust. All these things were going on together in our relationship and I suggest, all necessary for it to work well. In my example of Robert, who had an amputation without a major role in the decision process, it can hardly be said that he was fully in a position of trust, at least trust of a personal nature between us. It was not his choice to be admitted to our hospital. He didn't choose his surgeon. He was helpless in the chain of events beginning with his accident, retrieval and resuscitation and ending with his amputation. I was a stranger to him. The only trust he could perhaps have had in me was as a representative of an institution in which it might be reasonable for him to assume that I would act in his best interests. Even that assumes that I understood his best interests, although it's safe to say that I knew that he would most likely want to live and keep his leg. Even as a representative of the institution I was not completely controlled by the institution, as many decisions I made depended on my professional judgement.

Even though Robert was a stranger to me when I first met him, I knew that over a period of months I would get to know him well. Our team saw him regularly, constantly examining and discussing his progress with him, helping him towards recovery and a return to as full a life as possible. He was not a stranger when we bid him farewell and there are things I knew about him that many of his friends did not. While many patients are strangers, in the sense that we see them very briefly and relate to them only through a very small part of their lives, patients who have major problems, even in a large institution, frequently develop quite close relationships with the members of a medical team. Each stranger has the potential to develop a complex series of personal relationships with the individuals in the team looking after him. Every day until Robert left hospital and then on a regular basis as an outpatient visitor, we confronted the results of our care for him and were reminded of our responsibility for him. When the profession does this well consistently the community's trust is reinforced.

Corruption is essentially a breach of the trust that is given by the public to the holder of a public office. Whilst I do not claim that the profession of medicine is generally 'corrupt' in a criminal sense, Costigan[92] mentions features of a corrupt regime, which if used in a softer sense, might be found in any profession. Corruption occurs where:

> An organisation has built-in rules which retain the power

in a self-appointing cabal; secrecy, where a government or institution keeps its activities as private as possible and removed from outside scrutiny and accountability, where there is no independent mechanism in place to check the operations of an organisation.

Costigan was discussing the Olympic Organizing Committee and its lack of accountability and openness and points out that the I.O.C. assessed its own accountability on whether an individual within it had broken its own rules. Costigan's opinion was that the I.O.C. ought not to be judging its actions on rules manufactured within that organisation, but on rules that would be considered by others as acceptable and ethical.

Professions often do make their own rules and profess to be, and indeed often are, acting in the best interests of the community. If they operate only within their own rules, without listening to and accepting the ethical standards of the community as a whole, they can betray the community, because they are not able to be trusted to protect the community's interest as if it was their own. A profession, even when it is acting in its own self-interest, needs to know the best interest of the community and only the community can tell it that. To justify its actions a profession must be able to defend them publicly and be able to test these actions against the reactions of observers who are of normal intelligence and have a reasonable knowledge of the relevant facts. [93] Many professional bodies now have 'lay' representatives on the governing boards in an attempt to have more understanding of the broader community view. In spite of this their behaviour has not improved much.

A solid basis for institutional trust depends on a combination of the institution having rules and mechanisms for maintaining standards and the individuals within the institution having the capacity to honour those standards when decisions need to be made.

The idea of trusting an institution is a valid one and that trust is not necessarily a facade built to protect the institution, although institutions do have an interest in protecting themselves. A solid basis for institutional trust depends on a combination of the institution having rules and mechanisms for maintaining standards and the individuals within the institution having the capacity to honour those standards when decisions need to be made. In an ethical community, Hegel claimed, 'it is easy to say what a man must do', as he has specific duties laid out by that community. Hegel preferred to use the word 'rectitude' for the attitude to these duties, rather than 'virtue', virtue being that which he would equate to a demand somebody placed upon themselves, which would come into place usually only in circumstances when one obligation clashed with another. Hegel believed virtues are ethical principles applied to the particular. Hence they are something indeterminate and have 'their

Every profession needs to be aware of the interests and activity of all its members and be able and willing to challenge and correct, or even expel, individuals who do not acknowledge and practice the principles of that profession and at the same time act appropriately within their own personal ethical sphere. Neither a professional code of ethics nor personal ethical values are sufficient on their own, as both have to be applied together.

corresponding defects or vices, as explained by Aristotle, who we have seen defined each particular virtuous action as a mean between an excess and a deficiency'. An individual belonging to an organisation with an ethical order, has some freedom as an individual, because the basis of the ethical order, sanctioned by habit and principles, allows that individual to apply virtues appropriately. The rights afforded the professional individual are underpinned by duties they have imposed upon them by the ethic of that organisation. Hegel suggests that these duties may be easy as they are defined by the organisation, but the application of virtues requires some thought. To practice well a surgeon needs a clear professional structure with defined principles within which they are free to exercise their own judgment in the interest of the patient. This cannot work without an appreciation of common interests and in turn requires some knowledge of each individual's values and aspirations. Every profession needs to be aware of the interests and activity of all its members and be able and willing to challenge and correct, or even expel, individuals who do not acknowledge and practice the principles of that profession and at the same time act appropriately within their own personal ethical sphere. Neither a professional code of ethics nor personal ethical values are sufficient on their own, as both have to be applied together.

Chapter Ten: Emotions

At the end of the summer of 1993 Ken Poursain climbed over the railings of the Clifton Suspension Bridge in Bristol, England, intending to commit suicide. [94] A passer-by, Angela Stratford, stayed with him for three and a half hours and eventually coaxed him back onto the pathway. Prior to that episode Ken and Angela had not met, but they have since developed a close relationship they believe will last the rest of their lives. The friendship was not of a sexual nature. Ken wished to go back to his wife, as it was the break up in that relationship that precipitated his original distress and attempt at suicide. Angela said she did not think of Ken in a romantic sense but claimed, 'I'll always be there for him. If you save a life, in some way that life is yours. I really love him because he trusted in me.'

An examination of trust as a rational exercise suggests the trustee must have something to gain or achieve some self-gratification from the situation or there would be no reason for him to cooperate. A surgeon finds it easier to do his work if he is allowed to make some decisions for himself and receive a fee for his work, a confidence trickster to make money if he is trusted, and soldiers are more likely to survive if they trust each other. Angela Stratford appeared to have nothing to gain of a monetary or a physical nature. Angela may have had selfish motives for her actions, for instance being a trustee gives power and we can use this power to our advantage. A feeling of power is something most humans seem to value in itself as it fosters self-esteem. A trustee might also increase her self-esteem from the realisation that she is considered a person worthy of being trusted and therefore a person of some value. Trust can be an important part of personal relationships and there are not many warmer feelings than the knowledge that your friends trust you, as it can also be a very unhappy thing to find out that somebody no longer trusts you or considers you unworthy of being trusted. We may also have altruistic motives for being trustworthy as to do something for no other reason than to help another is a common and valued human attribute.

I was there for Alice, although I could not save her life. I tried my best. She understood that and comforted me. I cannot say I loved Alice because she trusted me, although love is a good word if it means a deep and profound fellow feeling. I was enriched emotionally by her and she helped me understand how I could be a better, more useful person. I too gained something of value for myself.

Angela Stratford was probably initially motivated by altruism when she stopped to talk to Ken on the Clifton Bridge as Ken was a stranger. Their relationship developed as Ken found that he could trust Angela while she talked to him on the bridge, showing that she cared enough about him as a human being and as an individual person to want to help him. It is unlikely that Angela only felt the need for some self-gratification and it seems very unlikely that she would have felt power over him. One could even argue that she might have found a greater feeling of power if she had suggested to Ken that, as his life was not worthwhile as far as she was concerned, he might as well jump. She could have played a significant part in what is one of the ultimate acts of power; that is being involved in effecting or hastening someone's death. On reflection, Angela considered she had gained something from the relationship and felt that Ken's trust her added a dimension and a meaningful extension to her own life. Angela loved Ken because he trusted and had allowed her to achieve something of value for herself.

I was there for Alice, although I could not save her life. I tried my best. She understood that and comforted me. I cannot say I loved Alice because she trusted me, although love is a good word if it means a deep and profound fellow feeling. I was enriched emotionally by her and she helped me understand how I could be a better, more useful person. I too gained something of value for myself.

Lawrence Blum[95] believes that, as each person is involved in a web of relationships, morality 'importantly if not exclusively consists in attention to, understanding of, and emotional responsiveness towards, the individuals with whom one stands in these relationships.' Care and responsibility do not need to replace impartiality and rational assessment, but rather complement them. A good example of this has been described in the difficult area of voluntary euthanasia. Advocates emphasise the importance of performing voluntary euthanasia within an established doctor–patient relationship. Van der Mass[96] describes how many respondents mentioned that 'an emotional bond is required for euthanasia, and this may be one reason why euthanasia was more common in general practice, where doctor and patient have often known each other for years and the doctor has shared part of the patient's suffering.' Critics might say that such a close relationship also increases the doctor's ability to unduly influence a vulnerable patient.

Blum[97] analysed the position of a teacher who gives special extra help to an illiterate boy. In this situation the teacher is not acting impersonally and has taken a compassionate role. This is not simply related to the teacher as a human being, but part of their response to the boy in their special role as a teacher. A teacher has certain values and ideals particular to their role.[98] The compassion and care that the teacher gives to their student appears to be distinct from the sort of compassion or concern they have for people in general. This is equivalent to my feeling that my surgeon should have some special compassion and care for me as part of their role. This is a role that is personal, although in a different sense it is also impersonal, as it is independent of the surgeon's personal characteristics and is an obligation of the role itself. I cannot see, however, how my surgeon could act independently of their personal characteristics, as they must have some idea of what it is to be compassionate and caring to be able to feel and exhibit these virtues.

Blum claims being a good teacher is more than just playing a role; it is being somebody who has a vocation:

> The notion of a vocation implies that the ideals it

embodies are ones that speak specifically to the individual in question. There is a personal identification with the vocation, that is, its values and ideals, and a sense of personal engagement that helps to sustain the individual in her carrying out the activities of the vocation.

A profession is a group of people who have particular knowledge and skills with social value and whose members have a sense of service. The professions claim a right to set their own rules and standards, based on their unique knowledge. They also hold special privileges in society. The professions set up fairly rigid internal structures and have specific rituals and symbols and tend to be pre-occupied with leadership. This makes them strong, but inclines them to isolation and self-interest. They are usually not particularly sensitive to outsiders, resist change and are hard to discipline from without. Therefore, they need to foster a much greater sense of vocation.

A vocation is a state of mind. It is also a group of people who identify with a common cause and feel they are part of something worthwhile. It has an ethos to which each individual contributes and from which each benefits. It is based on fellow feeling, caring and co-operation instead of rights and duties. There is an emphasis on inclusiveness, obligation and responsibility to others. It is less hierarchical and tends to be guided by individuals or groups who set a good example that others wish to follow. By its nature a vocation also tends to be weak and ephemeral and too easily controlled by others. Teachers need strong unions and doctors need strong colleges.

It is necessary to have surgical and other medical colleges. They perform important functions, including setting, teaching, examining, maintaining and regulating standards, dealing with government and other bodies and a wide range of administrative tasks. They have also lost their way, as in doing these functions we have lost much of our sense of vocation.

Not everybody can take up a specific vocation, as they may not have the personalities and attributes required for it. A person in a vocation must feel strongly about and identify with it and, whilst an individual in a vocation can have good personal values herself, she must also respond sympathetically to certain values outside of herself, those of her vocation, or she could not function within the vocation. Some good people will not necessarily make good doctors or teachers.

Whilst acknowledging that relationships in vocations, such as the doctor–patient relationship, are not the same as friendship, friendship does share with vocation a quality of having certain internal values, norms, standards, attitudes, and sentiments. Aristotle claimed trust is an essential part of friendship, 'nor can they admit each other to friendship or be friends until each has been found lovable and been trusted by each'. Thus betrayal is an ever-present possibility in any true friendship. A good friendship acknowledges this and uses trust as a measure of the importance of one friend to the other. For Aristotle it is important that each person has 'been trusted'. Not only should a friend be trustworthy but the friend also has to have given something of importance to the other to care for and the other willingly accept it. This, of course, could simply be a degree of dependence.

> And in loving a friend men love what is good for themselves; for the good man in becoming a friend becomes good to his friend. Each, then, both loves what is good for himself, and makes an equal return in good will and in pleasantness; for friendship is said to be equality, and both of these are found most in the friendship of the good.

In his list of things that may move men to anger Aristotle included signs of enmity or of disregard, particularly disregard that is 'disgraceful for them not to defend, such as parents, children, women and dependants'. He considered disregard as a proper cause of anger and lists, amongst other things, forgetfulness of names and thought, as forgetfulness arises through lack of concern, as a species of disregard. He also includes being belittled in front of others, ingratitude, and the actions of friends who do not perceive our needs. Whilst Aristotle does not describe these things in terms of betrayal, we would see as a betrayal the disregard for others whom we should protect and defend, as we might also a lack of concern when we have a particular relationship or obligation to someone.

Friendship does not have a definite structure and goals like a vocation as it allows for much more personal variability and individuality and is different in the sense that one doesn't have to be friendly, caring or compassionate towards everybody. Yet it is expected of a person within a vocation that they do care for all those they serve within that vocation. Thus, whilst the doctor–patient relationship is not one of friendship, it does share some of the virtues of friendship and the doctor has a particular duty to apply those virtues to all they meet within the relationship.

The idea of caring in a vocation implies specific types of caring depending on the vocation. A nurse, a doctor, an athletic coach or a lawyer will care for their 'charges' in different ways. This caring will involve different kinds of sensitivities and, to some extent, different virtues. In common is their regard for the overall good of those they serve. Blum also appreciates that there are distinct modes and sensitivities in caring that cannot be captured under general headings such as beneficence, benevolence and altruism. For instance:

> Being able to perceive that someone is depressed and knowing how to bring her out of it, is a different kind of quality to always being available to others when explicitly called upon. Yet both can be expressions of caring and both count as benevolence.

Being a good doctor implies that as well as having personal virtues there are virtues and emotions that are acknowledged as internal to the profession. Part of being a good doctor must include being part of a profession that acknowledges and applies those virtues. Not all members of a profession need to have all the same virtues, as the attributes of a good psychiatrist and a good pathologist are quite different. The profession itself must have and be able to apply through its members, those virtues necessary to serve the community. Ideally these general professional virtues should reflect those of the community itself, although sometimes a profession ought not to follow the community, as in the case of Nazi Germany. An exemplary profession might even lead a community to better human values.

Having a feeling is not sufficient to fully describe an emotion.[99] The feeling has to be about something. Cognition is the act or process of knowing. There is not always a particular kind of cognition when we have an emotion, as cognition may range over beliefs, thoughts and imaginings. With betrayal, the cognitive part may be an appreciation that something important has gone wrong with a trusting relationship and may be expressed like 'I gave you something I valued and you threw it away'. Someone can betray us without us knowing about it and we do not feel the emotions associated with betrayal without some belief about it. To have the emotions we need to believe that someone has betrayed us and feel associated affectivity. The affection leads to some reaction to the cognition. In discussing the 'affections' of the soul Aristotle[100] professed to be uncertain of their meaning but noted they are often associated with bodily changes:

> It seems indeed to be the case that with most affections, the soul undergoes or produces none of them without the body; being angry, for instance, and hoping, desiring and perceiving in general.

The various bodily effects that may exist range from non-felt changes, such as an increase in pulse rate or blood pressure, or noticeable changes, such as palpitations or dryness of the throat. The affectivity may be expressed by sadness, disappointment, despair or very strong feelings of alienation, dismay and anger. In discussing anger, Aristotle deemed it to be 'desire, accompanied by pain, for revenge of an obvious belittlement of one's self or of one's dependants, the belittlement being uncalled for'. This desire to act is the third element of emotion, which thus consists of three parts: cognition, affect and desire. In anger, 'the uncalled for belittlement of one's self' corresponds to cognition, the pain corresponds to affect and the desire is for revenge. The element of desire in emotion is usually expressed in behaviour, but need not always be so. Our reaction to betrayal might range from a mild unhappiness that is easily accepted, to wishing it had not happened, to recognition that being put in such a situation again would be unwise or to a profound desire to wreak some form of revenge. Any emotional reaction to betrayal must include some knowledge or belief about it. That is, you can be betrayed but, if ignorant of this, not feel betrayed. An act of betrayal may be no less real if you are ignorant of it, as it may still harm you, and others may notice and perhaps feel for you and wish to act for you.

Doctors do develop an emotional inhibition of their perception of pain in others; a two-edged sword, as whilst it allows them to work more dispassionately and make calmer, considered decisions, it also may reduce their empathy and compassion.

An attachment is some acknowledged relationship between people, such as friendship or love. It is difficult to give a non-emotional account of attachment that adequately captures the sense of loss we have when an important attachment is severed. If we do not suffer, the attachment was not very important to us; if we suffer a great deal it was very important. A sense of loss may be expressed through various associated emotions, including grief and anger. In a trusting relationship I expect my trustee to have a positive attitude to me and I would expect them to feel some emotion if they failed to look after me properly. I expect them to feel remorse if they betray one of my secrets or sadness if they tried hard to protect me but failed in spite of this. I would be disappointed if my surgeon did not feel some concern for me if my operation went wrong, even if they had done everything in their power to do the operation well. I would not expect surgeons to feel all my pain, and all pain of all patients, or very soon there would be no surgeons left as they would be too exhausted to continue. Indeed, Decety and others[101] found in a brain study that doctors tend to suppress the urge to empathise with other people's suffering. Shown images of people being pricked with various implements they responded differently to non-doctors, who had increased activity in their frontal and centro-parietal brain areas, by having no response in these areas. This suggests that doctors do develop an emotional inhibition of their perception of pain in others; a two-edged sword, as whilst it allows them to work more dispassionately and make calmer, considered decisions, it also may reduce their empathy and compassion.

There are times when we ought to have emotions, for instance, to be angry in certain circumstances, such as if we see a child being beaten. In close relationships we feel that our partner or friend ought to trust us and feel disappointed if they do not. Whilst we cannot be obliged to have certain emotions we may have an obligation to have certain emotional dispositions, and not having such dispositions can appear to be morally defective. Doctors should feel some affect or else patients will think of them as cold and unfeeling and not the sort of people they would wish to put their faith in. There is something in the relationship between my surgeon and I in which I expect some sort of reactive attitude on their part. I don't expect them to suffer as I do but I do expect them to acknowledge my suffering and to show some concern for it. This extends, I feel, beyond their obligation to treat me well physically and to relieve my pain as much as possible. I do not expect my surgeon to show pity for me, because that emotion seems to come from a distance, but to show compassion for me. I can forgive my surgeon if they make a mistake or an error of judgement but I cannot forgive them if I believe they do not care about me. This is more than I would expect from a merely contractual relationship and more than just relying on somebody to perform their function correctly and to the best of their ability.

I can forgive my surgeon if they make a mistake or an error of judgement but I cannot forgive them if I believe they do not care about me.

The emotions of remorse and guilt are central to a person who sees himself as a betrayer and can be overwhelming and persistent. A friend of mine, David, once said to me about his mother 'I have always felt guilty

I betrayed her'. David's mother had once said to him that if she became demented when she was old and feeble she would like him to kill her mercifully. The time came when she was indeed frail and demented but he did not kill her, not because he lacked the physical means, but because he was emotionally unable to do so. David felt he had betrayed his mother because he had not done something of great importance to her. I argued that he ought not to feel as though he had betrayed his mother as she was not justified in shouldering her son with a responsibility he did not want. Would David's mother still want him to kill her if she was aware of his emotional state, values and feelings towards her? She may not have wanted him to suffer in this way.

A relationship of trust implies some acceptance by the person being trusted of the responsibility of looking after the goods of the truster and it is the responsibility of the truster to be aware of this. I argued that David's mother ought not to have expected him to take on a responsibility he was morally and emotionally unable to perform. The emotion of guilt is particularly difficult to handle as there may be no outlet for the desired action that accompanies it. If the betrayer is not forgiven they can never resolve their own feelings and the long-term pain from this can be very damaging. Whilst many self-help manuals advise self-forgiveness this is not so easy.

When you are a doctor you must accept the burden of trust for all your patients. You make that choice yourself when you start your medical training and the only way to be absolved from it is to retire from the field.

In my view the person being trusted accepts some burden that can be onerous. Whether this burden is accepted voluntarily or not may depend on the circumstances. Most of us would probably like to be given a choice whether we are to be trusted with something, but perhaps particular roles, such as a between a son and his mother, suggests that trust is sometimes thrust upon us. David may have felt it was part of his unique role to acquiesce to his mother's wishes. Choices in trust may in part depend on values inherent in particular relationships and sometimes we have restricted choices as long as we remain in that relationship. We may leave the relationship, but on the other hand sometimes leaving a relationship may be seen to be a betrayal in itself. When you are a doctor you must accept the burden of trust for all your patients. You make that choice yourself when you start your medical training and the only way to be absolved from it is to retire from the field.

Sometimes we do not appear to be able to trust ourselves as most of us know situations in which we might be tempted to do something that we will later regret. Can I trust myself not to go to the casino and spend my pay packet, thus denying my family food for the week? What if I do go to the casino and against my previous better judgement lose the money? Unless I am a pathological gambler, who can think of nothing else but gambling, it is likely that subsequently I will have regret and self-loathing for my behaviour. I regret my moral weakness and I have not been true to what I might normally consider my enduring values. I think I can say I have betrayed my better self. It would be preferable if I distrusted myself and made sure I never went to the casino. Distrust can be a very reasonable and prudent defence against betrayal, even against one's self. If I do go to the casino and lose my money, why am I so upset with myself? I could say that this is just how I am and that is how I am expected to behave in such circumstances. Yet I do not think this way and I feel I ought to have behaved better and been more true to myself. Guilt may constitute a mechanism by which over time we can learn to be more trustworthy. A doctor may also need to trust himself to behave appropriately in certain circumstances. An example is if a doctor is tempted to have a sexual relationship with a patient or a teacher to bully a student. They need to know before they enter any relationship where there is unequal power that they are trustworthy and can trust themselves to behave appropriately. If they cannot, then they ought not enter into the relationship.

Our emotions play a fundamental role in our moral lives and 'without affectivity it is impossible to live a good human life and it may well be impossible to live a human life, to be a person, at all'.[102] An appreciation of the concept of betrayal emphasises the view that for satisfactory personal relationships to exist, particularly trusting ones, rational self-interest is an insufficient basis for these. Our emotions, at the very least, express the importance of many of the things that matter to us as humans. An understanding of the emotions associated with betrayal increases our knowledge of the concept of trust and, more importantly, our appreciation of the significance that trust has in the way we value our lives and how important it is for us to thrive.

If we use and monitor our emotions wisely we can improve all our

You cannot necessarily trust a professional; however, you should be able to trust someone with a strong sense of vocation.

relationships. By empathising with patients I have learnt to become a better person and a better doctor. When I was a student we had very little formal training in medical ethics but I was given a strong sense of vocation by my teachers and other role models. This has been strengthened over time by using both my reasoning and my emotional intelligence. The modern pre-occupation with professionalism, with all its dangers, and the formal structured teaching of ethics emphasising various formal principles of action, has diminished our sense of vocation to our detriment. You cannot necessarily trust a professional; however, you should be able to trust someone with a strong sense of vocation.

Chapter Eleven: The Emotions in Betrayal

A rational definition and analysis of betrayal cannot capture the nature of its intensity. An 'unemotional' analysis does not help us fully understand what it is actually like to feel betrayed, as a poem, play, novel or painting might do. An appreciation of the intensity of the human reaction to betrayal is necessary to expand our understanding of the nature of trust and its importance to us.

An illustration of the importance of trust and betrayal is found in Shakespeare's play *Hamlet*. One interpretation of the possible motives for Hamlet's actions could be that it is a guide to the affects of betrayal on a person and an illustration of the power of that emotion. The play concerns Hamlet's reaction to the death of his father and the subsequent hasty remarriage of his mother to his father's brother, who, Hamlet later discovers, has murdered his father. Neil Armfield[103] wrote of Hamlet: 'As much as anything else it seems to me that Hamlet is a study of trust, or rather, of betrayal.' He went on, 'In the absence of trust the mind and all our frames of reality spin out of control.' Trust is more than a medium for human interaction; it seems an essential part of human wellbeing. That is why, surmised Armfield, 'when surrounded by suspicion and in the dead centre of the play, Hamlet holds Horatio to him and declares with such relief what Horatio's trust means to him'.

Hamlet's reaction to betrayal is illustrated not only by his actions, but by the richness of his language and emotional response. If to some, Hamlet's reactions appear too violent and too extreme, it is important to place the play in the context of an Elizabethan audience. To them a marriage, no matter how hasty, to the brother of a deceased husband was considered incest. The marriage represents a strong blow to Hamlet, not just because of the death of his father, which might focus a man on the importance of human values, but because of a betrayal which makes him question the very worth of human values. The play reflects the human tragedy of a good, but complex, and in some ways frail person overwhelmed by circumstances. Through the course of the play Hamlet displays features that illustrate his reactions to his betrayal. After a period of depression and feelings of worthlessness come bitterness, uncertainty and a temporary period of inaction and shock. Hamlet then begins to react angrily and seeks revenge.

There seems little doubt that Hamlet feels betrayed by his mother Gertrude. His reference to 'incestuous sheets' and his comments on the frailty of women suggests a strong personal identification with how his father would have suffered had he known how little respect his wife had for his memory. The abruptness of her remarriage shocks Hamlet, not only because he feels that the memory of his father was not sufficiently valued, but also because Hamlet feels betrayed himself. Hamlet considers his mother ought to exhibit the virtues of motherhood, such as constancy, support, love and faithfulness. Gertrude has breached these virtues in dealing with her first husband and has engendered in her son insecurity and a fear of abandonment. As Judith Shklar[104] notes about the greatest of childhood anxieties, the fear of abandonment, that an action 'to reject a blood relationship for a new and alien association, or for none at all, is to deny the most elementary of social ties'. If Gertrude can betray Hamlet's father then she can, and has, betrayed him as well. Not only does he blame his mother, he is inclined to blame all women and his subsequent harsh treatment of his loving friend Ophelia may express this. Ophelia is a woman and like all women she will also betray him.

Sixty years ago Marion was seventeen years old when she noticed a small mole on her back. Conscious of her appearance she saw it as large and unsightly and persuaded her mother to arrange for her to see her godfather, Stephen, a leading plastic surgeon who was a close friend of her parents. Her mother, who had a flat brown lesion on her wrist, which she thought had been growing larger, also attended the appointment. Stephen examined both moles carefully, pushing them about and then photographing them from many angles. He said that he had time to excise only one of the moles and decided to do her mother's first, as Marion's was for 'cosmetic reasons' only. Sometime later Marion noticed the mole was bleeding and she saw her family doctor, who suggested she put a plaster on it and did not advise her to immediately return to see the surgeon. A family holiday further delayed her eventual return to see Stephen, who, when he saw the lesion, was visibly upset and agitated. The mole was a malignant melanoma and the diagnosis had been delayed. Marion overheard Stephen say to someone, 'If only it had not happened to Marion. Anyone but her.'

Marion had extensive surgery including removal of a large area of skin and muscle under the cancer and excision of lymph nodes and a large unsightly skin graft was taken from her upper arm. She spent much of the following year alone, depressed and despairing about what she saw as awful disfigurements. Eventually she worked hard to regain her strength and movement and returned to a normal life. Many years later she wrote to me:

> Did I feel betrayed at the time? No. I was incensed at the idea. This plastic surgeon, a very able man, had made an error of judgment. He was a doctor who was also a friend and no one, however lofty, can claim to be outside the very human possibility that errors will occur. He did his best, but he got it wrong.

Marion trusted Stephen on a number of levels. These may not have been obvious to her at the time, as trust is something we do not often think about, or at least not until it is too late. She allowed Stephen to look at her back and to touch, manipulate and photograph her mole. No matter how much she trusted Stephen as her family's close friend, a trust that had developed all her life as she learnt to know and love him, and he her, in these circumstances she also trusted him because he was a surgeon. She probably hadn't thought of that before and she slipped into the role of being a patient perhaps with some discomfort. Stephen the 'godfather' and Stephen the 'surgeon' were in some ways two different people. If Marion trusted Stephen as a surgeon, she did this without any previous experience of this side of him and probably relied on his reputation, her parents' faith in him and because surgeons are expected to behave in a trustworthy way. Then everything changed. Stephen's emotional reaction to his misdiagnosis and the delay in treatment was a complex one because of his unique relationship with Marion. She was not just any patient. It is difficult for us to imagine Stephen not caring for any young woman in such circumstances, but his position does complicate our reaction to his attitude to Marion and her subsequent feelings about what happened. Marion was vulnerable as she was young and inexperienced. Her description of the surgery and her reflections on her deformity show the major effect these had on her life and her view of herself as a young woman. This was something that really mattered to her and, in spite of support from her surgeon, and her family and her friends, she felt alone and despairing.

Marion is still incensed at the suggestion that Stephen may have betrayed her. Stephen probably felt very differently and he is unlikely to have thought it good enough to be 'very human' and was probably devastated that his faulty judgment let her down. Marion refers to it as an error of judgment, but she still thinks about it and wishes he had taken more care, although she does not recognise it as a feeling of betrayal. Her attitude to her father is different. He was always fiercely loyal to Stephen, as they had worked together during the war, and when Marion once complained to her father about Stephen's treatment of her she remembers him stomping off looking cross and not letting her say anything against Stephen. She felt betrayed by her father because she believed his loyalty should have been to her. Marion's mother was also upset because of her regret that she had had her mole removed first, which added to her natural fears for her daughter. Marion was always discouraged from talking about the whole episode and eventually gave up trying. As she grew older and talked to a friend with similar experiences to her mother she realised that her parents' reluctance to talk was probably because it was too painful for them to do so. Marion is able to understand and accept Stephen and her mother's actions but she has yet to forgive her father.

What stands out in Stephen's reaction to Marion is that he obviously cared about her and, no matter the result of his error of judgment, Marion has no doubt she was valued for herself. Although she was probably not aware of it, Marion was privileged. Imagine another young woman of similar financial and social means with a similar problem who went to see a surgeon she had never met before, who treated her professionally but not in a particularly friendly way and whom she felt had misdiagnosed her condition and delayed her treatment. This surgeon, although not dismissive, does not show any emotion or remorse for what has happened. What would this young woman say about her surgeon? How much more likely is she to feel betrayed and not to forgive? It would be understandable if she decided to sue him to exact some recompense. It is another thing again for a young woman who lives in a poorer part of the community, who presents at a public hospital and only sees junior medical staff in the clinic and never sees the same person twice. If she is lucky she meets the consulting surgeon briefly as he has a cursory look at the lesion. A form of consent is sought by a junior medical officer and she is presented with a long complex document, which she is asked to read in front of him and which she feels she has not had time to comprehend and think about. She does not fully understand but she has to sign before anything will happen. She is not given the opportunity to see the consultant after the surgery and feels that nobody really cares about her or her fate. It is not difficult to compound these problems with the possibility that the pathology report may be mislaid, misunderstood or not fully interpreted by junior staff. Add to this the possibility that when she eventually gets to definitive treatment, the operating session is cancelled for reasons that are not made clear to her. If something goes wrong she will feel angry, powerless and despairing. How a person reacts to a situation depends on her circumstances. With exactly the same lesion, a similar delay in diagnosis and treatment and the same outcome, Marion accepts and does not blame her surgeon, although later she does wonder about it, another woman feels betrayed and is able to act upon it and gain some financial recompense and yet another woman is left feeling angry and helpless.

Twenty-five years later Marion was married with three young children. When she decided that she had had enough of hairdressers catching their combs in a lump on the crown of her head her doctor sent her to see another specialist, as Stephen had retired. Marion informed the specialist of the melanoma excised when she was 17. He examined the scars of the earlier surgery and pronounced the lump to be a 'harmless naevus'. He injected some local anaesthetic into the area, gathered up the strands of her hair, still attached to the mole, lifted the whole thing into the air, cut around the lesion and, with a pair of scissors, chopped the hair off a couple of centimetres above it and dropped the lot into a specimen bottle. He then sutured the wound and sent Marion home. After later removing the sutures he did not arrange another appointment.

Six months later, when the area hadn't healed and was still sore, Marion's mother noticed that another mole had appeared in the wound and that it was black. Marion saw another surgeon who excised a sample for biopsy, which indicated that this was, as suspected, a second melanoma. A large divot was cut out of her scalp leaving a bald patch. Another time of anxious waiting followed. The specialist who originally excised the mole was informed and he rang her in the evening at home and told her that he had contacted the pathologist to whom he had sent the original specimen and had been told that the slide had 'gone missing'. He was sorry, very sorry.

Marion felt helpless and angry and believed this doctor had betrayed her trust by not shaving the area to enable a clear view or sending the specimen to a pathologist. She felt he was covering up the possibility that he had performed an inadequate excision and had acted without proper care and didn't want others to know about it. Marion believes his protestation that the slide was lost was deceitful but she has no proof of this. She has been left with a feeling of violation and impotent rage. Her description of the surgical procedure graphically illustrates both the symbolic importance of her physical integrity and her actual physical sensations and reactions. She still feels and sees the strands of hair that were crudely used to separate the lesion, which was then dropped, as if carelessly, into a bottle.

Surgeons are usually allowed to intrude upon a willing patient's physical integrity and consent is given for them to do so in the belief that it is for a greater good. This doctor, however, was careless. He did not take the lesion seriously and had no understanding of Marion's underlying fears about the nature of the lesion. He either failed to ensure that the specimen was properly reviewed by a pathologist or had no record or recollection of that review. His failure to follow up appeared to her as though she'd been abandoned and he may have deceived her. His later expressions of sorrow were not accepted by Marion as sufficient reparation for his guilt. This was a doctor who ought to have known more about his patient, who ought to have taken more care with the procedure and who ought to have followed up with kindness and consideration. Marion feels betrayed by a man who was a special person, a trusted doctor, who did not treat her with sufficient understanding and imagination and who had no consideration for her as an individual.

It may appear astonishing that the experience of a patient with her doctor could possibly be compared with the enormity of Hamlet's feeling of betrayal. At first sight Gertrude's actions appear much more hideous than that of Marion's specialist, yet the strength of the emotions Marion felt were also totally overwhelming: she seethed about it and lay awake at night thinking about. Hamlet's depression and feelings of worthlessness are no different to how Marion felt when the doctor she put her faith in treated her so carelessly. She was afraid of the possible consequence of an early death and thought about ways of exposing the doctor's treachery and harbored a wish for vengeance. Hamlet rages against his mother because he feels she owes him personal regard and love and rages against women in general, because he sees her as a representative of the necessary role of women to support family structure and security. Marion feels similarly about doctors. As well as their obligation to individual patients, she believes doctors also have, as part of their role, an obligation to support social and family structures and personal security. Marion describes feeling disappointed in and depressed about her lack of judgment leading to her misplaced faith in the man, helpless anger at the perceived injustice and a deep feeling of loss. If one doctor could treat her like this, could not they all? She lost faith in the whole medical profession in the same way Hamlet lost faith in all women.

Much like Marion, Hamlet is depressed, believes he is a victim, is bitter and has a sense of loss associated with feelings of foolishness, powerlessness and anger. After a period of uncertainty Hamlet attempts to re-establish himself by taking action against the betrayers and seeks revenge. During this time he also starts to develop some acceptance of the situation, particularly as his mother shows considerable remorse. However, the tragedy is never resolved for Hamlet, as his uncle perpetrates a further betrayal and the action ends, not with Hamlet's re-establishment, but with his death. Hamlet was a powerful man and was able, eventually, to take action against those he believed had wronged him, although these actions were destructive, both to him and to others. Many others, including the ill and disadvantaged, may not be able to take action after a betrayal and their sense of loss and helplessness, like Marion's, can continue unabated.

In the play Hamlet asks a group of travelling actors to perform for him. To illustrate his talents one of the players performs a piece by Virgil, the author of the *Aeneid*. The *Aeneid* is a tale of the siege of Troy and what follows from the Trojan viewpoint. The actor tells of the grief of Hecuba at the slaughter of her husband Priam on the battlefield. During the speech the actor's eyes fill with tears. Ironically, Hamlet finds it monstrous that this player, 'in a fiction' could mimic such a strong emotion when Hamlet's own real emotions must be so much stronger:

> What's Hecuba to him, or he to Hecuba,
> That he should weep for her? What would he do,
> Had he the motive and the cue for passion
> That I have? He would drown the stage with tears.

The sufferings of Hecuba can give us more insights into betrayal. Martha Nussbaum's examination of the Greek playwright Euripides' *Hecuba*, written in 424 BC, further illustrates why the betrayal of trust matters so much to us. The play is about events surrounding Hecuba, the defeated and enslaved Queen of Troy, following the fall of Troy to the Greeks, via the ploy of the wooden horse, after a ten-year siege. Simply put, the play is in two parts, the first being where Hecuba's daughter,

Polyxena, is sacrificed on the tomb of Achilles after the fall of Troy. Hecuba accepts and copes with this great loss partly because of the strength of her character and her belief that Polyxena is genuine when she states she would rather die than live as a slave. Hecuba believes Polyxena has been treated according to her worth. The second half of the play is about Hecuba's reaction when she discovers that her special friend, the man she trusted above all others, has murdered her son. Hecuba had trusted Polymestra, an old friend and ally, with her youngest son Polydorus to keep him from harm during the war. Polymestra betrays her by throwing Polydorus off a cliff so that he may keep his fortune. Hecuba is unable to cope with the death of her son because this has been perpetrated by her most trusted friend. Hecuba lives in a society in which ethical commitments and standards are human constructions. In this world, human agreements, practices and values are the ultimate authority for moral norms. As even the Gods exist only within this human world, if convention is wiped out there is no higher tribunal to which she can appeal.

If the most important relationships can be corrupted, then all relationships can be.

If Hecuba's best friend cannot be trusted with her most precious possession, her social structure is stripped away from her and, like Hamlet, she 'spins out of control'. She contrives to blind Polymestra and kill his sons. An important distinction that Nussbaum makes is that the betrayer is a special friend, who of all people has the most obligations of care and protection, perhaps like Hamlet's mother. This ought to be a relationship that is inviolable as it is fundamental to Hecuba's view of interpersonal relationships. The loss of trust is particularly damaging because Hecuba does not see the relationship with Polymestra as being like other relationships, such that might be between lovers or ordinary friends. If the most important relationships can be corrupted, then all relationships can be and once the deepest trust is seen not to be trustworthy everything collapses into complete disorder. For Hecuba, it is not only the outside world that becomes disordered, but also her view of herself. The basis of her existence as herself, that is, the recognition of her self-worth by the person whose stability and trust is most important to her, has gone. The only way Hecuba sees to fill the void and attempt to restore order is to take revenge. She replaces the previous value of the network of trustworthy human beings with solitary, power-seeking, vengefulness.

The second half of *Hecuba* illustrates that if morality is only a system of human practices, these practices can be defiled. It is possible for this sort of moral society to cope with individual breaches of trust, if in general all others conform, but if the whole social fabric goes and nothing external to it exists to hold it together, individuals are no longer able to trust each other and become intent on self-protection. This is the position Hobbes[105] takes in the *Leviathan*. Hobbes believed it was inevitable that men would break their covenants unless there was some strong external force to bind their promises. Hobbes' world was not so dissimilar to our own, in which many of our moral values no longer come from a theological view point but depend on human virtues and social values. Without an external, inviolable, incorruptible, moral structure the loss of any internal structure that has developed through the customs of the community is likely to affect the stability of any individual involved.

Whether or not you believe in the divinity of a God you are still liable to a profound betrayal by those who profess to know the truth, who base their actions on this assumed truth and who are not to be trusted with their stewardship.

Such devastation is, of course, not confined to non-believers in a divine presence. The victims and families of paedophilic activities of priests and others have been equally disturbed by their betrayal, both by the individuals and by the priestly hierarchy who failed to recognise, accept and take steps to fix the problem. This was compounded by the church denying and covering up the transgressions and avoiding or delaying compensation. Whether or not you believe in the divinity of a God you are still liable to a profound betrayal by those who profess to know the truth, who base their actions on this assumed truth and who are not to be trusted with their stewardship. These assumed truths are not necessarily divine ones, as all professions and other groups who claim to have a special type of knowledge, and for which they may claim special privileges, risk betraying those over whom they hold power.

Chapter Twelve: The Trustee

I once believed I had betrayed Mary by being careless and not fully checking all her particulars before operating on her. With much trepidation and guilt I came to her bedside, confessed and said how sorry I was. 'That's ok,' she said. 'I trust you.' She trusted me, continued to believe in me and accepted my mistake. She insisted I keep treating her and later asked me to operate on her again. It was not a question of forgiveness, she said, but of continuing faith in my character and goodwill. I was not so sure.

The old song, *I would be true, for there are those who trust me,* by Harold Walter, implies that if we are trusted we will feel some personal obligation to those who trust us and suggests that trust is not merely a device for cementing some certainty and commitment in relationships, but imposes an obligation on the trustee that goes to the core of his character. Mary reminded me how important the good parts of my character were to her and how essential it was for me to be true to these. I had to try harder to be worthy of her trust.

Trust is not merely a device for cementing some certainty and commitment in relationships, but imposes an obligation on the trustee that goes to the core of his character.

In a commercial transaction it may be sufficient for us to obtain reliable and understandable information about fees and profits. In other situations, however, we can get understandable, comparable and reasonably objective information about the quality of performance and yet feel we need to know more about the character of the people we are dealing with. When I used to take my children into their school classrooms it was not just the quality of the work produced that impressed me, but all of the teachers' skills that made the classroom a good place to be. The good teachers were warm, kind, encouraging and caring, qualities much harder to measure than literacy and numeracy. Schools are relatively safe places, but there are always risks. Despite the disclaimers and waivers presented to be signed by administrators and teachers I usually trusted the teachers to look after the children as well as they could. I made personal judgments about the attributes of individual teachers, but I also trusted them because they were professional teachers whose role it was to care for children. A good teacher has certain values and ideals that are particular to her role as a teacher. The compassion and care that the good teacher gives to her student may be additional to and, in a way distinct from, the sort of compassion or concern that she might have for people outside the teaching relationship. This is a role morality that is independent of, and in addition to, the teacher's personal characteristics as it is an obligation of the role itself.

In the first chapter I described the difficulties my surgical colleagues and I were having answering charges of bullying and sexual harassment and suggested one problem was that we did not really see the problem. Iris Young[106] argues that our society is dominated by the values and ideas of the privileged and the values of rich societies have been assumed to be universal values. The values of a surgical group are usually those of the senior members. New trainees are often selected, probably unconsciously, because they appear to the seniors as fitting a proper mould and then, as they live and grow in the culture, take on more and more of its character. Young argues that we should question values we think as 'given' and think more of injustice as oppression. People are likely to be treated unjustly for reasons such as their race, colour or gender. In an environment where people do not recognise oppression, the use of reason to remove bias becomes too abstract, as the powerful do not see the problems of the oppressed because they are blind to them. The powerful need to listen to those they may not hear at first, as justice requires us to be able to hear a cry of distress and to respond to it. Theories of justice that depend on rational principles don't help us much as they don't touch us or inspire reaction and, whilst reason can clarify issues, we must be able to develop a sense of justice based on listening to others who we may be unconsciously oppressing. Our junior colleagues, of whatever gender, race or other characteristics, should be able to trust us to listen more carefully to their concerns and to open our closed eyes.

We have not yet looked deeply into the mirror or, more appropriately, into the eyes of our juniors to learn how we should behave in order for them to trust us. I have not forgotten what I saw in the eyes of the junior registrar I betrayed. Martha Nussbaum also discusses the importance of mutual self-recognition to individual awareness. She writes of the 'image of the reality of the connection between me and you' metaphorically reflected in the eyes of another. If the other sees nothing I am nothing. Plato developed this theme in *Alcibiades*,[107] where he claims that 'just as self-seeing requires seeing one's own image in the eye of the beholder, so self-knowledge concerning things of the soul requires knowing oneself in another's soul.' To know what self-consciousness is like we need to be able to observe another self-conscious being and we cannot develop self-consciousness in isolation, for self-consciousness grows out of a social life and a child growing up in isolation from other self-conscious beings never develops fully. Each person needs another person to establish his own awareness of himself and requires from the other an acknowledgment or some recognition, as a person's self-consciousness is threatened by the existence of another person who fails to acknowledge him as a person. Hegel[108] believed that self-consciousness has itself for its object, but to form a picture of itself, it requires some object from which, by contrast, it differentiates itself, as 'I can only become aware of myself if I am also aware of something that is not myself'.

Our own sense of self-worth is fostered by the emotions others have towards us. If others appear to have a benevolent concern for our welfare and express this with kindness and warmth this affirms that we matter: If people do not display positive emotions towards each other, our sense of self-worth is seriously threatened, for 'the feeling that everyone around one is indifferent towards one is truly demoralising.'[109] An emotional sense of our own and others unique importance is fundamental to our sense of wellbeing.

At its best, the profession of medicine shares with teaching the idea that its members may have ideals and values that go beyond the specifications and duties expected of other professions. If I need to have a heart operation and have managed to organise my finances so that I can afford to choose my own surgeon, I will assess them in a number of ways, not the least of which will be their technical competence and the reputation of the hospital in which they work. Yet I will look for more. I feel that my surgeon should have some particular care for me, as a human individual, apart from their technical ability and clinical judgment. I would like my surgeon to have some sense of vocation. I expect my surgeon to have personally embraced the values and ideals of a good surgeon and for them to use those values to both guide and sustain them. If my operation goes wrong and my life is in danger I would also like to know that, whatever the outcome, they will care for me to the limits of their personal and surgical abilities. I would expect them to go home that evening tired and emotionally drained. As much as they can, I wish to trust them to deal with my needs as if they were their own and to deal with them in the light of their own best knowledge and conscience. How a surgeon should relate to their patient is not necessarily overtly stated, as there is assumed some sense of obligation of one person to another and of the surgeon to their patient. Certain rules of behaviour may start simply as matters of convention or convenience but over time can take on the characteristics of a moral obligation as these rules are internalised. The community assumes that surgeons will follow rules particular to their occupation, whether stated or not, and it is to be expected that they have incorporated these rules into a commitment that has become part of their own sense of vocation.

At its best, the profession of medicine shares with teaching the idea that its members may have ideals and values that go beyond the specifications and duties expected of other professions.

The good surgeon, in an Aristotelian sense, practices all the appropriate skills until they mastered them, but they may not become trustworthy in a professional sense until they have reached a degree of practical wisdom or clinical judgment and internalised certain moral obligations.

This requires them to have the ability to make independent decisions in particular situations, based on their own experience and judgment, and to apply them in a trustworthy manner. Aristotle suggests that the only person who could judge a surgeon appropriately is another surgeon. No one but another surgeon can fully appreciate the skills and mature judgment of their peers. We cannot, as a community, however, accept only the judgment of a surgeon's peers, as we know that professional groups have a tendency to look after their own interests and we all have various biases. These biases are often unconscious. Trustworthiness is difficult to assess and in part will depend on the personal experience of the patient as well as the measurement of outcomes. This is a good reason to record, analyse and respect the experiences of patients as part of our training and continuing education.

Whilst it is clear that the truster usually has a significant emotional involvement in a trusting relationship, less has been said about the feelings of the trustee. It may be instructive to look at the doctor–patient relationship from the point of view of the surgeon. Why might surgeons wish to be trustworthy? Trustees of any sort are vulnerable to loss of friendship and abuse from others and even to having legal action taken against them if things go wrong. It is necessary for a trustee to understand, take care of and to make decisions for the truster and it might be a lot easier, if it were possible, to have some type of formal contract so that trust is not required. When we are trusted we have a burden placed upon us, as whilst the truster takes a risk in trusting, at the same time they place a responsibility upon the trustee, as now we are expected to care and act well towards them, simply because of the very idea that they do trust us. In being trusted, the trustee is expected and must try to be trustworthy. As Mitchell[110] states:

> To understand trust from the perspective of the trusted is to understand that trust is more than a device for reducing transaction costs or worldly complexities, for smoothing the way of business, for building successful economies or even coherent societies. To understand the importance of being trusted is to understand the way in which the responsibility for trust reposed can affect character.

Being a trustee may impose a major burden of time, effort and emotion; yet the realisation that they are being trusted can make a person want to be trustworthy. Mitchell uses the example of some characters in a Steinbeck novel (*Tortilla Flat*, 1953), who are moved to act honestly, against their original intentions, by the simple trust of an acquaintance. The fact that he trusts them changes their attitude to him and forces them to examine their own consciences and they begin to sympathise with him. Their characters are changed as they respond to the emotional challenge of recognising the needs of a fellow human; indeed, eventually it seems to them that they have no choice but to be trustworthy and so they are. In the musical hit, *Les Miserable*,[111] Jean Valjean has been released from prison but cannot find employment and reverts to a life of crime. Whilst being sheltered by the Church he steals some silver. He is caught and arrested but the Bishop forgives him, secures his release and gives him a further two silver candlesticks, exhorting Valjean to use the silver to reform and become an honest man. Valjean does this successfully but is pursued and eventually discovered by an avenging policeman, Javert. Valjean escapes and later has Javert at his mercy but releases him, thus completing his redemption. Javert later commits suicide as he is unable to reconcile his commitment to doing his duty as a policeman and being merciful.

We have all had similar experiences of being trusted, although, alas, we do not always respond well. If we recognise our failure, we often feel guilty and resolve to do better in the future. Over time we may notice an improvement in our character. Mitchell argues that the moral psychology of being trusted, in that it helps to create trustworthiness in people, makes personal trust a rational process. A sense of vocation, with its inbuilt moral structure, can reinforce this character building and lead a teacher or a surgeon to see being trustworthy as an end in itself. Javert, however, a strict Kantian, is unable to do this, as whilst he may value trust, it is subordinate to his duty. In this sense he is true to his professional values, as the values of a policeman are rightly different to those of a schoolteacher or a doctor. This does not contradict either a Kantian categorical imperative or Aristotle's position that some things should not be considered as a mean between two extremes and are just wrong. Javert has contradicting professional and personal values and pays a high price for this. This is not a unique situation, as doctors and teachers may have similar conflicts, for instance over abortion or teaching evolutionary theory. We may sometimes feel we have no choice but to choose between one position and another. This places a great burden on the trustee as they may have to choose between continuing to be trustworthy and their personal moral position. It may be difficult or impossible to reconcile their duty to the truster and to their own beliefs and, in some cases, one or the other will suffer. Most likely both will suffer, as whatever decision is made will lead to deep feelings of compunction.

There is a reverse process: not being trusted can lead to untrustworthiness. We find it difficult to live or work with someone who does not trust us. If our actions and motives are constantly being checked we eventually lose confidence in the relationship and become unable to make appropriate decisions. At the same time we may lose confidence in ourselves, as we see the other person does not honour our integrity and we begin to doubt our own self-worth. We can respond with anger and a sense of loss but eventually this cools and may be replaced with indifference. Once we become indifferent and cease to care about the other we stop acting well towards them and we become untrustworthy. Failure to trust may eventually lead to loss of trustworthiness by the trustee. Untrustworthy behaviour leads to further lack of trust and a lamentable situation exists with a vicious downward spiral that is hard to break.

The intensity of the emotional reaction to a betrayal of trust must suggest that we feel something valuable has been lost. The value of trust, reflected in the intensity of our emotions around betrayal, is related in a complex way to how we feel about others and ourselves. We value both a person who is trustworthy and one who is able to trust. We believe a person who cannot trust to be misanthropic and a poor member of society. These values reflect the way we think about our place in society and our relationship to the world in general. Being trustworthy and able to trust contribute value to society as a whole because they increase social cohesiveness and allow us to achieve things in small groups that otherwise could not be done. Fighting in a war safely and successfully and playing in a premiership sporting team both require comradeship, understanding and the ability of each member of the team to trust and be trusted by others. Captains of both can give guidance and instruction and can establish principles of action, but on the field it is the relationship that is built up between the players and their acceptance of individual responsibility, as well as the team's ability and strategy, that make them successful.

> *On the field it is the relationship that is built up between the players and their acceptance of individual responsibility, as well as the team's ability and strategy, that make them successful.*

Early in Raymond Chandler's seminal detective novel, *The Big Sleep*,[112] Philip Marlowe meets Carmen Sternwood, the daughter of the man who is about to become his client, in the expansive entrance hall of General Sternwood's grand home.

> 'You're awfully tall,' she said.

> Then she giggled with secret merriment. Then she turned her body slowly and lithely, without lifting her feet. Her hands dropped limp at her sides. She tilted herself towards me on her toes. She fell straight back into my arms. I had to catch her or let her crack her head on the tessellated floor. I caught her under her arms and she went rubber-legged on me instantly. I had to hold her close to hold her up. When her head was against my chest she screwed it around and giggled at me.

> 'You're cute,' she giggled. 'I'm cute too.'

Carmen expects Philip to catch and hold her, thus ensuring immediate physical intimacy, and he does so. She gambles, correctly, that his immediate reaction will be to save her from harm, even though, as he does so, he is aware of the awkwardness of the situation. His action immediately places him at a disadvantage as the butler enters and finds Carmen in his embrace. Carmen has trusted Philip's human instincts and used them to her advantage. The truster has used her own power to control the trustee. Carman becomes the more powerful person by making herself vulnerable and forcing Philip to act out his natural disposition to catch a falling human. Most people would have instinctively caught her, no matter who she was. A fully rational and knowledgeable Marlowe may have let her fall, and thus avoided the physical trap she set, and in that sense he would not have betrayed her as the illusion of trust she creates is false. Marlowe is betrayed by Carmen because his actions are those expected of a normal, responsible person. It is Carmen who tears the fabric of society. The momentary power is hers although she quickly loses it as he does not trust her again. The effects of her actions are to Marlowe's permanent disadvantage as to external appearances he has taken advantage of her. The fabric of society is difficult to repair and the shreds will always be weak and may never be recoverable unless it is pulled apart and rewoven anew. This may be not so easy, as we now know something about the other that we did not before and this will be woven into the canvas. Betrayal is about abusing social and personal expectations and tearing social and interpersonal bonds. It is also about wielding power inappropriately over the disadvantaged or dependent, whatever their apparent strengths.

The trust and betrayal between Marlowe and Carmen appears trivial or nothing compared to that of say the violation of a long-term marriage, but it is nevertheless very real to the participants and the readers of the novel. It serves as the basis of many, if not all, human relationships. The worker who claimed his employer betrayed him by locking him out when he was on strike may have felt his employer owed him something, perhaps to care for him or honour a contract, even though he may be seen by his employer as behaving badly. This suggests the employer should understand and respect his point of view, although also suggests that the worker should respect that of the employer. Each protagonist is wary of and influenced by the potential power of the other, which, they suspect, may not be used to the best interest of all. As trust thrives on goodwill, its lack may lead to betrayal. If it becomes a power struggle the ultimate winner may lose the trust of the loser with consequent long-term problems, which, overall, may not be in the winner's long-term interest.

A functioning community develops a sense of order, which in a Hegelian sense is associated with a commitment, sometimes unconscious, to community cooperation and commonly shared norms. This order comes from constantly practicing good social behaviour and Hegel comments:

> When a father inquired about the best method of educating his son in ethical conduct a Pythagorean replied; 'make him a citizen of the State with good laws'.

Fukuyama recognised this as a commitment to a general social structure. We expect these structures to be permanent and cannot live without some general expectation of the order of things. This expectation, however, is probably based only on an inductive premise that such things are likely to happen. As time passes we normally become more certain that things will happen but become less certain if the behaviour of people around us is inconsistent or misleading. What is certain, however, is our need to act as though there is some structure in our lives. Force of habit allows people to feel as though the social structure is real and to behave as if there is a solid basis for it.[113] Aristotle[114] has made the point that even the law itself depends on the habits and the support of the community: 'The law has no power to secure obedience save the power of habit and that takes a long time to become effective'.

The difficulty of everything requiring a contract is that it does not allow any activity outside of the rules.

Those who are fearful of trusting do not have faith in others' commitment to social cohesion. If people are unable to trust then they may either have to withdraw from full participation in society and individual relationships or they can attempt to make the bond stronger. One way of making the bond stronger is to have formal rules and laws, which substitute bolts for bonds. This is equivalent to having relationships as covenants or contracts. The difficulty of everything requiring a contract is that it does not allow any activity outside of the rules. This may lead to significant restrictions in our everyday lives and in the choices and options we may wish to make. It is difficult to imagine any human life flourishing without the ability to make some non-contractual decisions. Forcing people into contracts may encourage them to be deceitful in order to achieve their own advantage. A society that depended only on contract would be a narrow, uncaring one in which we might be even more vulnerable to the deceit of others, because there would be no reason to show anyone goodwill. As Lao Tzu wrote in China in approximately the Sixth Century BC:

> When a society needs rules of conduct for relationships, hypocrisies and deceit will emerge. The situation here has reached a lamentable stage.[115]

If the bonds of society fail, where there is absence of trust, there is nothing left as a basis for human relationships and people will become isolated and perhaps, like Hamlet, 'spin out of control'. The Greek historian Thucydides[116] described such a situation after the destruction of the town of Corcyra by the Athenians:

> An attitude of perfidious antagonism everywhere prevailed; for there was no word binding enough, no oath terrible enough to reconcile enemies. Each man was strong only in the conviction that nothing was secure; he must look to his own safety and could not afford to trust others.

A hospital can appear trustworthy and keep reasonable standards by regulating the behaviour of its employees, but decisions have to be made that depend on the knowledge and integrity of the individuals within. In some circumstances individuals will have to be trusted to do certain things. How they react will depend on their own character and training. To appear trustworthy and to encourage people to trust them, it is not enough that a doctor, as Machiavelli[117] recommended, should only 'appear a man of compassion, a man of good faith, a man of integrity, a kind and religious man'. Machiavelli reasoned that:

> Men in general judge by their eyes rather than by their hands; because everyone is in a position to watch, few are in a position to come in close touch with you. Everyone sees what you appear to be, few experience what you really are.

To become a good trustworthy doctor a student needs to practise being trustworthy and to be able to act on behalf of, as Aristotle taught, 'the right person, to the right extent, at the right time, with the right motive, and in the right way' and 'That is not for everyone, nor is it easy'.

Doctors need to be truly trustworthy. Any illusion of trustworthiness will be seen to be false if the doctor does not have those virtues necessary to act fully in the interests of their patients. Hegel argued that a person in an institution has to be more than a mere follower of rules, he has to be able to make good decisions for others, and 'a doctrine of virtues is not a mere doctrine of duties'. An institution cannot for long sustain the illusion of trustworthiness unless its members are genuinely trustworthy. Machiavelli[118] eventually realised this and warned that a state (or a hospital for that matter) might not be able to function if 'by ill chance the populace has no confidence in anyone at all, as sometimes happens owing to its having been deceived in the past either by events or by men'. The publicity generated by the complaints of deceived patients may eventually undermine any public trust the hospital once had. To become a good trustworthy doctor a student needs to practise being trustworthy and to be able to act on behalf of, as Aristotle taught, 'the right person, to the right extent, at the right time, with the right motive, and in the right way' and 'That is not for everyone, nor is it easy'.

Chapter Thirteen: Forgiveness and Justice

Harry was a 70-year-old man who needed a total hip replacement. Before the surgery I discussed with him the common complications of the operation, including death from a blood clot in the lung or a heart attack. He took the information in and signed up for the operation. Unfortunately, he had an unexpected complication from a technical problem during the operation and the result was a sub-optimal procedure. Crestfallen, I told him later what had happened. 'That's ok, Doc,' he said. 'You are more worried about it than I am, you said I might die, this is nothing compared to that.' He later had a successful revision operation and never once complained.

> Son, thou art ever with me, and all that I have is thine.
> It was meet that we should make merry, and be glad: for
> this thy brother was dead, and is alive again; and was lost,
> and is found.

Luke 15: 31–32, King James Version of the Bible

The parable of the Prodigal Son describes the reaction of a father welcoming a son who has returned after abandoning his family, going far away and wasting his inheritance. The son asked for his inheritance early as he wanted to enjoy it whilst he was young and active, but unfortunately he spent it all on having a good time, finished with nothing, and was hungry and poor. This prodigal son asked his father to take him back and help him, which the father did with joy. Another son, who had stayed, worked hard and helped his father, was angry at his father's reaction as he felt that the prodigal did not deserve such a welcome and it was unfair on him. The father replied that he loved his faithful son and would give him all that he had, but he would also forgive and welcome the son he thought he had lost with open arms.

Forgiveness can recover something that appeared irretrievably lost and allow an important relationship to begin again.

I have always liked this parable as it powerfully illustrates how forgiveness can recover something that appeared irretrievably lost and allow an important relationship to begin again. Lessons have been learnt and the most important values established. The father's forgiveness is unconditional and he rejoices in this. There is no blame or recrimination as the prodigal is accepted as he is just as, in a way, Harry accepted me. Later, father and prodigal son may have sat down and discussed his behaviour and how each had thought about it. Perhaps an even better relationship was forged. It reminds me of how Salman Rushdie[119] describes the reconciliation between a man and his grown up son. He expresses the need for a father to admit his vulnerability and be able to share his weakness with his son in the hope his son will be able to uncover and share his.

> You left me as a boy and you have come back to me as a man. Now we can talk as men of manly things. Once you loved your mother more. I do not blame you. I was the same. But now it is your father's turn; a turn I should more rightly say, for us. Now I can ask if you will join your force to mine, and hope to speak freely of many hidden things. There is at my age a question of trust. There is a need to speak my heart, to unlock my locks, to unveil my mysteries. Great things are afoot.

The prodigal's father does not need his son to admit his vulnerability. He sees it, accepts it and forgives. There is no certainty that the prodigal may not go off on his own again and hurt his father in other ways, but he will always know he matters. The faithful son asks questions that we would all ask. Should the prodigal acknowledge his foolishness and perhaps work to make up for his profligacy? Should the father accept some responsibility for giving a son his inheritance too early? What of the justice of the situation? The faithful son could reasonably claim to be disadvantaged by his father's actions and feel he has been let down or even betrayed by him.

In Rushdie's novel the father is seeking and wishing to share something with his son. Because the son has returned and been accepted they can both acknowledge their love and need for each other and open up to share their deepest thoughts. Through forgiveness and acceptance both benefit as the act of forgiveness has liberated them. In Shakespeare's play *The Merchant of Venice*, Portia says to Shylock, who is seeking his just reward of a pound of flesh from Antonio:

> The quality of mercy is not strained, it dropeth as the gentle rain from heaven upon the place beneath: it is twice blest: it blesseth him that gives and him that takes.

Mercy cannot be forced, but when given, benefits the giver and the taker. Yet we are sympathetic to the faithful son and in other situations believe certain actions are unforgivable. Adam Smith[120] argued that we are free to be kind to others, yet cannot be forced to be kind, although kindness to others is often praised. However, we can be obliged to be just towards others, as a violation of justice is an injury, which can be disapproved of or punished. Hence being beneficent, which cannot be forced, is quite a different thing to being just, which can be subject to obligation. In the same way, whilst we can be grateful for the beneficence of others, we cannot be forced to be grateful. Gratitude may be freely given whereas the acceptance of rights may be taken without thanks. The prodigal's father chooses to forgive his son but the faithful son may consider his father is obliged to treat them both justly.

Plato[121] argued that justice couldn't only be giving someone what is theirs, as doing so may affect others adversely. An example he uses is that if someone asks for the return of a weapon, it would be unjust to give it to him if you knew that he intended to use it to kill another. In this case we make a judgment on the appropriateness of our actions, depending on how we see it will affect others as the benefits of what we owe various people may have to be balanced against each other. Plato concludes that justice is related to the functioning of the whole community and a just society consists of individuals being able to properly complete their required tasks, depending upon their place in the community. It is not just to forgive a surgeon who abuses their trainees by making excuses for them, such as, 'he is doing it to toughen them up' or 'he is stressed', as this will adversely affect those who follow and thus lead to the overall harm of all trainees. It also entrenches similar behaviour in all surgeons as they see it as an acceptable part of their role. This is not to ignore that there may be a necessary toughness inherent in the role of a surgeon, or that it can be stressful, but that these things need to be managed so others are not harmed.

Hobbes believed that there was no such thing as justice, only equality achieved through power. To survive, individuals had to become part of a power structure capable of fighting off the voracious advances of the rest of humanity. Charles Eccles-Smith, who suffered cognitive impairment following surgery, was relatively powerful, being a member of the profession that betrayed him, yet nevertheless responded to his betrayal with a period of depression and bitterness. He attempted to reassert himself and right the wrong he felt had been done to him by educating others through publishing an article about his experiences. Martha Nussbaum suggests that actions like Charles' reflect more than an attempt for personal rehabilitation, they are also an attempt to re-establish the social fabric as 'The logic of revenge sets the world to rights, most of all by making it reveal the hidden nature of its former crimes'. Justice requires bringing things out into the open so all can see.

Sometimes the search for revenge can become an obsession for an individual and as Nussbaum writes, 'Revenge takes over the entire world of values, making its end the one end.' Mrs Whitaker and Dr J.'s patient were able to show very clearly that they had suffered harm and they were able to express their bitterness and anger by blaming the doctors involved. They used the power of the legal system to obtain some recompense and re-establish themselves. I imagine one of the costs of this to them would have been a prolonged period of legal action in which the ill done to them was constantly in their minds and their anger continually reinforced. It would have been better for all if the problems had been openly discussed initially, the transgressions discussed and the actions understood. Then there may have been no need to seek revenge.

Whilst human experience suggests that Hobbes in some ways is right, his outlook was too bleak. Adam Smith recognised the general fellow feeling we have for any person, even a stranger. A sense of what is good for others and the mutual benefit for all humanity creates the greatest benefit, or utility, for all. One of the great criticisms of utilitarianism, however, is that in maximising the community's overall benefit, there is a risk of trampling the interests of less powerful or socially isolated individuals. John Stuart Mill[122] sought freedom from the tyranny of powerful individuals and organisations and oppressive social practices. He saw the conflict between social utility and individual freedom but believed the free actions of well-cultivated individuals was the basis of a good society, providing their actions did not harm others. It is important to recognise the difference between Mill's freely acting and feeling personal individuality, and Kant's autonomy obliging the individual to follow rules that all the members of a rational community would agree upon.

Justice can be defined as treating people with equal respect as autonomous moral agents, irrespective of their social position, race, colour or gender[123], but neither utilitarian nor social contract theories seriously consider an individual's sense of obligation to others, even to the point of putting their rights or interests before their own. Plato[124] argued that individual integrity, the idea of being just for justice's sake, is good in itself as 'the just life profits a man'. Carol Gilligan[125] challenged what she felt was an essentially male view of moral development, which is based on theory, rights and justice, and replaced it with the idea that a person's life is enriched by co-operating with others, as we belong to each other and by caring and co-operating we make the world a better place. A just world becomes one in which we maximise the number of people able to have and enjoy a life in which they can fully develop and exercise their capacities and express their needs, thoughts and feelings.[126] One way of doing this is to develop a more Hegelian view of justice in which each individual within the culture sees themselves fully contributing to and benefiting from a common goal.

A just world becomes one in which we maximise the number of people able to have and enjoy a life in which they can fully develop and exercise their capacities and express their needs, thoughts and feelings.

My experience is that most people find it hard to forgive, whatever the slight, but to forgive a betrayal is especially difficult. This is understandable as a betrayal suggests we were worth little or nothing to the betrayer. To forgive we not only have to recover from the betrayal, we must regain our own sense of worth. It may help if we try and understand the betrayer, their motives, feelings and actions. If we can put ourselves in their shoes and believe they now see how we feel and acknowledge what they have done to us and regret it, we can begin to forgive. In his analysis of 'Tit for Tat' Singer suggests, whilst it is important to be aware of the past behaviour of others and to be suspicious of their motives if their behaviour has been bad, there is no way of changing a bad relationship without somehow being able to forgive and start again. Although we must be careful, there is real value in 'beginning or resuming a cooperative and mutually beneficial relationship with those who have, in the past, been uncooperative'. Singer believes that rational behaviour of this type strengthens social relationships and, like Hume, believes a sympathetic partial relationship with others reinforces the strength of this 'rational' behaviour.

In 2006 the American Psychological Association produced a brochure to complement a workshop on forgiveness.[127] They describe forgiveness as a process that involves a change in emotion and attitude regarding an offender. This is a voluntary decision to forgive, in spite of the victim's full recognition that he or she deserved better treatment. It requires letting go of negative emotions toward the offender and results in a decreased motivation to retaliate. Forgiveness can occur in the absence of reconciliation, just as reconciliation can occur without forgiveness. Forgiveness can be a one-sided process, whereas reconciliation is a mutual process of increasing acceptance. Forgiveness is different from condoning, that is, failing to see the action as wrong and in need of forgiveness, and excusing, which is not holding the perpetrator responsible. Forgetting is not enough, as forgiveness is more than just forgetting about the offence, it requires a change in the truster's affective response.

Looking back, I regret the times I have *not* forgiven more than those when I have. There are those whose poor behaviour to me I have forgiven and I continue to value their friendship, although sometimes with reservations. Those who I was not able to forgive were lost to me. Some of my best friends are those who were able to forgive me or I them. Perhaps we should expand Aristotle's opinion that friends have to have trusted and been trusted by each other, to sometimes include those who have forgiven and been forgiven by each other. A strong friendship is one able to cope with many human frailties. We would be at times uncertain and cautious, but we would not be alone.

A strong friendship is one able to cope with many human frailties. We would be at times uncertain and cautious, but we would not be alone.

Sometimes it is not that the person being trusted has failed but that the person who is trusting has made an error of judgment. The truster has made a choice not to be independent. The truster may be at least causally and, possibly at times, morally responsible for any transgression and betrayal by the trustee. In the same way a person might deliberately make themselves vulnerable and dependent by trusting another to gain an intangible something that makes them feel more complete and valuable. The doctor–patient relationship is one between unequals and it is hard to blame the patient if they are betrayed, although sometimes, if they have made a decision to trust when they could have known more or ought have been more prudent, then perhaps it is possible to do so. In Marion's account of her experience as a teenager, Stephen's reaction was clear to her as he was upset and agitated and expressed his dismay that it was not 'anyone but her', and he worked hard to get the best possible result for her, in which he was successful. Marion, in spite of her initial protestations, has been left with a perception of betrayal by Stephen, something she has had difficulty defining, and yet she gives the impression that she is, perhaps, defending him too strongly. How much is this a justification and support for her own trust, which she may have blamed herself for accepting too blindly, thus denying her own responsibility, although she was young and asking too much of herself? She is much more definite about her father, who she did believe had betrayed her by appearing to defend Stephen when she thought he should be more concerned about her. Eventually, Marion has accepted Stephen's actions, as he openly showed he cared about her, and forgiven her parents, as she has realised she must have mattered a lot to them and the whole episode had become too painful for them to talk about. She has not forgiven the doctors who later treated her indifferently, probably lied to her and did not diligently examine and keep the pathology specimen or follow her up. But she has remained angry and has difficulty in forgiving others.

Most of us respond to betrayal with anger. The longer our outrage lasts the longer we remain angry and when we are angry we cannot consider forgiveness. We can remain angry for very long periods, sometimes for the rest of our lives and long periods of anger are bad for us. There is some evidence[128] that people who can unconditionally forgive others, that is they do not need the other to apologise and promise not to do it again, live longer than those who cannot forgive. It is postulated that those who harbour resentment and grudges, continually nursing negative feelings and anger, keep their stress levels high and perhaps this shortens their lives. Being compassionate to the betrayer may have other benefits, as there is now some evidence from brain imaging that being compassionate stimulates the same pleasure centres associated with the drive for food, water and sex and may be protective against disease and increase our lifespan.[129]

Hannah Arendt[130] articulates the importance of forgiveness to the betrayer if broken relationships are to be restored:

> Without being forgiven, released from the consequences of what we have done, our capacity to act would, as it were, be confined to one single deed from which we could never recover; we would remain the victims of its consequences forever.

The hardest person to forgive is yourself, doubly so if your self is entwined in your work. To forgive another is to see them, make a decision and move on independently. To forgive yourself does not allow you to move on so easily, as the betrayer is within you and always present in your memory. I remember the times I betrayed others more strongly and for longer than I did when others betrayed me.

Most of us want to hear an apology and a promise that it will not happen again before we can even consider forgiving a wrong, but if we do forgive under these conditions, it is conditional on the apology. The physical and emotional damage to ourselves has to be restored and this can be helped by an apology and perhaps some financial or other reparation, but the most important restoration, that is the loss of our self-respect, must come from within ourselves. It is better for us if we can forgive unconditionally by discarding our anger and accepting the wrongdoer, whatever their faults or motivation. It is often our own anger, rather than the betrayal, that harms us most. If we can't forgive we remain subservient to the betrayer's actions and can never completely restore our own self-esteem and equanimity. This may require us to attempt to understand the betrayer and his motivation and actions.

Forgiveness may require having understanding sympathy and compassion for the betrayer.[131] The betrayer themself may be angry, jealous and insecure and this may underlie all their actions. This does not mean forgetting the betrayal, as the betrayer needs to know the damage they have caused and possibly requires help to overcome their own lack of understanding. Forgiveness may require re-assessment of the betrayer so it does not happen again, unless we choose to take the risk again. This suggests two attitudes to betrayal, one in which we forgive but do not forget, and protect ourselves by avoiding situations that have led to betrayal in the past, and another where we forgive and allow the betrayer fully back into our lives and accept the vulnerability. Tit for Tat does not work fully unless we do the latter but implies we have accepted as genuine the promise of the offender not to do it again, acknowledging the possibility he may not live up to the promise, even with the best of intentions. At some stage with a repeat offender we may eventually decide that enough is enough. A deeply felt betrayal is not so easy to forgive.

With forgiveness both the betrayer and the betrayed are freed to re-establish relationships and get on with life. According to Brene Brown all humans thrive on connection[132] and fear being rejected and shunned by others. We all live in a state of vulnerability and those who are able to cope with this appear to have a strong sense of worthiness, that is, a strong sense of being loved and belonging. Brown calls these people 'wholehearted'. They have the courage to tell their story openly and truthfully, admit to imperfections and have empathy and compassion. Wholehearted people embrace vulnerability and Brown asserts we should let ourselves be seen and live and love without guarantees. Wholehearted people may be able to forgive unconditionally.

We all have difficulty coming to terms with our isolation and our lack of true understanding of each other, whilst at the same time we emphasise and value our uniqueness and autonomy. Our emotional dependence on each other and our need to love and trust is opposed to the realisation that no state of being appears to be able to blend our isolation and dependence into some harmonious whole. It may be that trust is a way of overcoming our sense of isolation and, in a peculiar way, making ourselves vulnerable to others reduces this sense. Thus a decision to forgive may be based on the realisation that there may be nothing on which to base forgiveness, because essentially there is nothing to forgive, as we are each searching for a connection that has no tangible substance, but one nevertheless that somehow has power and importance to us. Forgiveness has real benefits for the forgiving victim. It aids psychological healing and improves physical and mental health, restores a sense of personal power and helps bring about reconciliation between the offended and offender. To be compassionate to the offender the victim has to work through their own pain and anger, to reflect on their own past offences, learn from the experience and see themselves as more than just a victim. Gandhi thought that only strong people could forgive, but it may be that it is the act of forgiveness that makes the victim strong.

Gandhi thought that only strong people could forgive, but it may be that it is the act of forgiveness that makes the victim strong.

The betrayer also has a responsibility to help the victim heal. To do this they have to first recognise themselves as a betrayer. This is difficult as we are often blind to the effects of our actions and tend to down play them when they are brought to our attention. Often we are never aware of our betrayals and it may require the strong efforts of outsiders to wake us up. If we do recognise a betrayal we need to reflect upon it, acknowledge our role, openly and personally seek out the victim, admit and apologise for our actions and ask for forgiveness. It is probably wise to eventually try and forgive ourselves, as ongoing guilt, and the anguish that can bring, is bad for us as well, and may inhibit our own attempts to fully re-establish trust. It is important to believe you can and should be trustworthy once more. Within institutions it is important that it is the individual betrayer who approaches the victim, as a general, seemingly remote apology from an organisation is never enough. The modern idea that many failures of trust are due to system failures within organisations, and that individual people are not responsible, is unlikely to cut it with the individual victim. It is hard to forgive if you do not know who has betrayed you.

Portia's speech preceding her assessment of the quality of mercy in *The Merchant of Venice* advises, 'Though justice be thy plea, remember this, that in the course of justice none of us shall see salvation' and suggests that mercy is the better solution. Can a patient forgive an untrustworthy doctor? This is not a question asked of a genuine mistake or misjudgment, where there may be nothing to forgive, but where the doctor has not honoured his patient's integrity. To do so the patient either must have a strong sense of wholeheartedness or have had their integrity restored in some way, as forgiveness must come from a position of equality or it is no more than submission. As healing is a major tenet of medicine, it follows that if a wronged patient is to be healed, it is part of a doctor's role to help their patient through their reaction to the betrayal. This means the doctor has to openly approach the patient, explain themselves, seek to be understood, listen to the response, express sorrow and ask to be forgiven. This is what my college is now doing for those trainees we have damaged. But it is not enough for the college as a whole to apologise for the individual offenders. They must be brought to do it themselves in full understanding of the damage they have done. In an emotional and litigious environment this may be very difficult to do and may require considerable outside mediation.

It is for individuals to forgive, if and as they choose, and for the surgical profession to be always just.

The members of an offending surgeon's profession, however, cannot afford to forgive them, as their actions strike at the profession's very being and the safety and integrity of all those they serve. It is for individuals to forgive, if and as they choose, and for the surgical profession to be always just. If the profession is itself unjust and we cannot recognise and remedy injustices that are part of our culture, we can expect and must accept that more powerful outsiders will do it for us.

Chapter Fourteen:
Trustworthiness

I began my journey as a young boy in a suburban railway train who lost his simple faith in the care and goodwill of girls and proceeded over a lifetime to perform acts of betrayal myself. I never lost my belief in the value of trust and lived in the hope that one day I would reach my ideal of being truly trustworthy. Having failed in the latter, I turned to the study of forgiveness and found some solace there, but could not escape the burden of guilt and the stern eye of justice. I now understand the importance of empathy and compassion and the absolute imperative of trying to be honest and trustworthy. As difficult as it is to honour and maintain trust, trust, by holding us together through its tenuous bond, may be the only thing that can give us happy and fulfilling lives.

As difficult as it is to honour and maintain trust, trust, by holding us together through its tenuous bond, may be the only thing that can give us happy and fulfilling lives.

Trusting relationships between doctors and patients may, at their best, reflect a deep human commitment which, whilst less than love and different to friendship, is in some ways expected to be more solid and more reliable than those two. The effect of betrayal on the doctor–patient relationship has an importance that can be at least as profound as, and sometimes greater than, that seen in more personal relationships, and that loss of trust can have devastating and lasting effects on the patient. Medicine seems to offer a distinctive source of hope because trustworthiness is essential to its nature. Without faithfulness these human activities would not be what they are. Betrayal in these contexts, therefore, is especially destructive of trust and the moral balance is correspondingly more difficult to restore.[133]

Each generation has different problems to solve and within each generation we come to terms with one problem only to find another has presented itself. Over time our answers to each of these problems changes. My mother, a nurse, had no difficulty believing it was acceptable to lie to patients for their own good. My parents, frightened and weary of war, believed that the use of nuclear weapons was appropriate and I as a young doctor had no idea of the concept of informed consent. Now we debate the correct age to resuscitate very premature infants, the ethics of gene therapy and when to withhold expensive and possibly futile therapy from the elderly. As I write this we are trying to understand and control bullying and sexual harassment. Within these topics each situation is different, the answers rarely certain and unanimity uncommon. Teaching ethics is not like teaching anatomy, mathematics or French. There is no constant, firm basis of fact and each problem has to be thought through anew. Because each situation is different, choices difficult and outcomes uncertain, very few of us are ever sure our actions are correct and if we are certain we are probably deluding ourselves. It is in this environment that doctors and their patients exist, each being all too human and prone to error. We have no choice but to trust the goodwill and integrity of each other, knowing that sometimes this will fail. To help others effectively it is necessary to be trustworthy.

If I am to be worthy of trust I must be able to try and put myself in another's position, assume their values and aspirations and act on these, as well as I can, as I sincerely believe they would wish me to act. The trusting person gives unto my care something that they value because they cannot, or choose not to, look after it themselves. In a mutually trusting relationship I agree to act in their best interests and they accept that I may have to make decisions about how to do this. I need to know something of the value of what matters to them and they expect me to have some personal obligation towards them. They may be prepared to and perhaps ought to forgive me if their person or possessions are damaged in spite of me acting with due care and goodwill. They possibly may forgive me if I have been careless or thoughtless, providing they accept my human frailty and contrition. They will find it very difficult to forgive me if I have been disloyal, dishonest and uncaring and have not honoured their personal integrity. Sometimes they may choose to forgive me unconditionally, for their own or both our sakes.

In many modern societies there are no fixed rules for solving moral dilemmas, nor indeed, is there a coherent general moral philosophy. I live in such as society. Most decisions we make, however, use one or more of the following maxims:

> **An individual person is important in themselves.**
>
> **Individuals are normally responsible for their own decisions.**
>
> **We should apply the same rules to ourselves as we do to others.**
>
> **We should think of others as we do ourselves.**
>
> **We should try and maximise the common good.**

All these maxims are contained in most religious and secular orthodoxies, although the emphasis and application varies and many add theological or sociological exhortation and support. If we are to practice the above maxims it may be easier if we add a few simple rules such as:

> **Do not tell lies.**
>
> **Do not kill.**
>
> **Keep secrets.**

Yet we can all think of extreme situations where it might be appropriate to lie, kill or reveal secrets and only a few of us would never do them given the right circumstances. If we find rules hard to apply we can think of a few principles to use, such as:

> **Respect autonomy.**
>
> **Be just.**
>
> **Do good.**
>
> **Do no harm.**

These principles may appear easier to use than firm rules, as they are not absolute. Yet they are harder as well, because when conflict exists it is not easy to appreciate another's autonomy, what is just in a particular situation or how to avoid some harm. In respecting one person's autonomy we can be unjust to some and harm others, and in being just we can restrict someone's autonomy.

A good society needs to have people with the knowledge, virtues, skills and experience necessary to appropriately apply any maxim, rule or principle in the course of their daily lives. Those are the characteristics of a good citizen. As well as needing to be such good citizens, doctors have particular responsibilities requiring a high degree of commitment to these ideals. Our society expects us to maintain this responsibly and allows us certain privileges and powers in order to do so. The doctor–patient relationship can be strengthened by commonly available communal ties, such as fiduciary duties and contracts, although both these in their own way are somewhat antithetical to the relationship, as they tend to restrict our ability to make the choices that may be essential for a good outcome. Important is a Kantian ideal that honours the patient as a person of value in themselves and who is always to be treated as an end and not a means, as is a model that emphasises preserving the patient's emotional integrity and their feelings of self-worth. These need to take into consideration the overall good of the whole community and the maintenance of a just society. They are difficult ideals to maintain in day-to-day relationships and a doctor–patient relationship based on trust, in which the doctor learns and practices these ideals in a trustworthy way, will serve patients best. This is essentially a virtues-based model that also relies on the sensible application of principles, an understanding of the consequences of one's actions and a duty to treat the patient as an end in themselves.

A rational assessment of trust is not sufficient in itself to explain its scope and importance. Trust does not work from the point of view of self-interest alone and requires individuals to learn to co-operate. A strategy such as 'Tit for Tat' does work, but needs the first move to be one of trust, which requires no more than some expectation of reciprocal good intentions. Humans often trust strangers without any sound knowledge of the other's motivation and goodwill and without considered rational thought. Trust is different to reliability because we believe the trustee has a special requirement to care for us and what we value and to take some personal responsibility for these.

Trust is critical to the wellbeing of both personal relationships and society as a whole. Anything that increases this, such as good personal relationships, human sympathy and altruism, appears to strengthen trust by making us more certain of the bond that holds the structure together. This bond is not a tangible thing that can be seen and measured but is real to us within our commitments to each other. A contract also increases cohesiveness, but relies on powers imposed from outside the relationship and reduces the participants' internal necessity to behave honourably and may thus diminish the bond between people. The bond in trust expresses our commitment to the structures of society and interpersonal relationships. A reciprocal commitment from others to the structures strengthens the bond, yet we cannot totally rely on it as we know from experience that others do not always pledge themselves as we would wish. A strong general commitment can survive some infidelity if the bonds between us are strong. Repeated or overwhelming breaches may destroy the bond, the structures will dissolve and chaos may result. To re-establish trust we usually require an acknowledgment of the betrayal, expression of contrition and a resolution to do better. We resist cheats and find it difficult to forgive even though a just forgiveness often creates the opportunity for a better outcome.

To have insight into another person's cause requires knowledge, empathy and understanding and to deal with it requires goodwill, imagination and integrity. The trustee's judgement and actions may, in retrospect, turn out to be different to that which the truster wished, but as long as the trustee has acted in good faith with the truster's interest at heart, then the trust has not been violated. In such a case the truster may have an obligation, due to the nature of the trusting relationship, to forgive the trustee if things go wrong.

Many patients are rendered powerless and deeply distressed and angered by a betrayal. They are often not able to right the wrongs and regain their self-esteem. The medical profession tends to look after its own and it can be quite difficult for a patient to achieve recompense for any harm. Taking legal action is a major stress for most people and it is expensive and often unsuccessful. It is important for individuals to be able to re-establish themselves and gain some form of empowerment in their lives. The doctor who betrays a patient has a responsibility, as part of his role as a healer, to assist in the patient's recovery. It is very important for patients to have a forum, such as a patient advocacy commission, that encourages them to express their emotions and to come to some terms with their treatment. The medical profession has on the whole been reluctant to accept and cooperate with complaint commissions and doctors have a not unnatural desire to protect themselves from criticism. This is to the detriment of the patients they are pledged to support. If these commissions were wholeheartedly supported by the profession, and open enough to allow the full expression and discussion of the various problems, this would enable patients to achieve some re-establishment of their own self-worth and hopefully to begin to trust again.

Patients have responsibility in the doctor–patient relationship and if they consent to treatment when in possession of adequate information, they should accept any problems that occur within those agreed parameters as part of their responsibility when they made an informed choice. It is not easy for patients to make informed decisions because it is difficult to grasp the meaning, language and presentation of the information they require. An obligation for doctors to communicate well, rather than to fully disclose, should be considered and the quality of this communication assessed. Whilst adequate, understandable and well-presented information is likely to significantly reduce the risks of misunderstanding, it is still probable that patients will have to take some things on trust. The necessity for trust should be recognised in the law and, although the nature and uncertainty of trust would make this difficult, taken into account if the doctor honoured the interests of their patient as if they were their own. The trustee has to be able to justify their actions. The patient may accept this and be able to forgive a doctor for well-meant but incorrect choices. This can only be achieved within an open truthful dialogue.

Understanding our emotional reactions to betrayal will guide us how to respond to people who have been betrayed. Patients can quickly lose faith in doctors who fail to live up to the virtues expected of them. A loss of faith in the character of a person who is trusted, particularly if it is in an important relationship, can severely affect an individual, not only in that relationship but in all trusting relationships and lead some to believe that all relationships are insecure. In the doctor–patient relationship trust can be enhanced by educating and empowering patients so they understand their condition and are able to take some responsibility and be involved in their own care. Patients should be educated in the values, virtues, powers and faults that the doctors they need to trust are likely to have. This would lead to the most satisfactory form of informed consent. Doctors have to be trained to be good at their jobs in the fullest Aristotelian sense and must work in an environment that encourages virtues such as honesty, understanding and compassion as well as knowledge and technical expertise. The profession of medicine must be seen as one that will not tolerate their members lacking these virtues. It is imperative to have some basic absolute rules and a general commitment to truth telling, confidentiality and individual freedom.

We often have no choice but to trust institutions and the individuals within them. To be trustworthy an institution needs to have a solid understanding of its duties and the will and power to enforce them. Institutions are not usually good at this as they tend to look after their own interests. Individuals within an institution have considerable independence and need the necessary virtues to work honestly and well. Various forms of discrimination, harassment and lack of respect for the less powerful are common and are often not recognised by those who should know better. Those subject to the power of an institution should have a right to monitor it and if necessary seek to change it.

The medical profession has its own difficulties maintaining trust. Once one problem arises and is addressed another soon surfaces. How quickly and thoroughly these concerns are addressed often depends on the publicity generated and the embarrassment felt. In my own college the most recent concerned bullying and sexual harassment. One complaint centred on the college being dominated by Anglo-Saxon males whose values perfused the culture of the college. This was probably true when I joined but is slowly changing, although the culture is strong and pervasive and does tend to envelop and convert newcomers to the old ways. Over my time the sons of European migrants became dominant and later the children of Asian migrants have been influential and now women are slowly finding a stronger place. Each generation gradually influences the culture, although not as radically or quickly as people outside the profession would like. It is not easy to break into an established culture and in doing so we tend to be absorbed into it and thus take on its characteristics. Established within the culture we can no longer see with an outsider's eyes. Once, when a problem arose my college tended to react defensively then later we would have set up an internal committee to investigate and report, and even later we included a selected outsider to give 'balance' to the proceedings. To our credit, with the latest problem, the sexual harassment of our junior trainees, the committee consists of a majority of knowledgeable outsiders. Perhaps every institution should set up a completely independent and powerful 'Board of Good Behaviour'.

Perhaps every institution should set up a completely independent and powerful 'Board of Good Behaviour'.

The idea that trust should be a rational process equates with professionalism and the need for contracts, rules and social sanctions. The concept of vocation can include these whilst emphasising ideals, virtues and duties that are internal to the individuals in a vocation and are of that vocation. The individual becomes part of that vocation and shares the values expressed by it. Thus professionalism should be a lesser part of the healing and caring vocations. A successful caring community allows its individual participants to act freely with the necessary virtues of the role they play within the community, and which they have internalised from the values of that community. The caring community is successful if it also shares the ideals and values of the general community it serves. This implies a constant conversation between the vocations and the general community, each listening to the others views. The carers serve and may advise the general population but they are ultimately responsible to them and can never be self-sufficient.

In the final analysis the maintenance of the web of expectations and commitments resides in the hands of those involved within the trusting relationships. This is where expectations of behaviour assume a moral importance as, if we return to Hegel's original definition of trust, one which I have found no reason to fundamentally dispute, a trustee has to respect me and look after my interest as though it were his own. What matters to me has to matter to the trustee. Respect for autonomy is particularly important in the medical encounter as often the doctor and patient are unequal in power and the patient finds it difficult to express and implement what their autonomy means to them. It is inevitable that in some circumstances doctors will have to make decisions affecting a patient's autonomy without a clear idea of the patient's best interests.

A trustworthy person needs to have sufficient empathy and sympathy to recognise and care for the needs of others, especially when they are less powerful and vulnerable. A good doctor does this with compassion and with a sense of vocation. Both the trustee and truster may be enhanced by a good trusting relationship and damaged when it fails. The betrayed believe they have not been recognised and honoured as important in themselves and are personally diminished. For the betrayed to recover they have to re-establish their self-respect, often by some apology, recompense or revenge. The most difficult, but perhaps the best way to recover, is to forgive the transgressor. Forgiveness needs to be tempered by a sense of justice as forgiveness too lightly given may disadvantage others and allow cheats to prosper.

The betrayed believe they have not been recognised and honoured as important in themselves and are personally diminished.

The strong emotions displayed in betrayal emphasise how important trust is for humans to flourish. We are all isolated, vulnerable, individuals, striving for independence yet constantly needing to belong and interact with others like us. We seek those who recognise and value our own selves and who wish for us to recognise and value them. No law or social convention can enforce this and it is probable that trust, for all its dangers, is the only way we can achieve it.

Trust is an unspoken bond between us all, which, if broken, leaves us dismayed and angry. Without this trust, all relationships are without true worth. Trust does more than make worthwhile things flourish; it is essential to their growth and stability. A total loss of trust is devastating as there is nothing left to keep us together and all relationships seem meaningless. We think others ought to help create and preserve the social fabric and expect everyone should behave with consideration for others. This is not quite the same as the Golden Rule of doing unto others what you would have them do to you, although this is part of it, nor quite the Kantian maxim that you should only act if you are prepared to accept that the principles you are following should be applied to all. You should act as well as you can to maximise the best interests of others and expect they should do the same to you. This is the basis of a successful trusting relationship and depends on the goodwill, imagination, understanding and empathy of all involved. It is a version of Tit for Tat in which there is an expectation that it is more than a game and each party genuinely cares for the integrity and welfare of the other.

The emotions associated with betrayal reflect our dismay at anything that appears to be a loss of commitment to the forms of social order. The emotions are also our reaction to the failure of somebody to recognise and act on our unique personal individuality and worth. Any individual within the social order is expected by the other members to give some commitment back to that social order and not to live in isolation from it. Betrayers either do not see or ignore this social bond. This may be reflected in our belief that betrayers ought to gain some insight and express their contrition by emotions such as anguish and shame. If they fail to do this, and even sometimes when they are contrite, we often want to take strong action for recompense or revenge.

The trustworthy doctor comes with a sense of vocation. A vocation is something important, more important than any individual.

A good doctor will be one who promotes the patient's interest as well as possible. They will need all the virtues and experience of a person of practical wisdom to achieve this. Whilst there is a need for some basic rules of behaviour and principles of action, the essential task in training good doctors will be to impart in them the virtues of a wise, trustworthy physician. These virtues are different to those required of a lover, a friend, a lawyer, an accountant or an architect. They include virtues common to all good living, such as veracity and good will, but also specific virtues related to knowledge and technical skills and the cardinal medical virtues of empathy and compassion. Doctors who do not have these virtues place the entire community at risk, for if the trust of the people is lost, no doctor can work effectively. The trustworthy doctor comes with a sense of vocation. A vocation is something important, more important than any individual. It is this that gives life and meaning to professionalism and stops it from being a self-seeking charade. By fostering and developing the vocations of caring and healing we will become more trustworthy.

Take care of the bond of trust, because it is all that we have.

Notes

1   Things may be different now as my surgical college runs a course entitled *Communication Skills for Cancer Clinicians: Breaking Bad News,* in which surgeons are guided through 'real life' scenarios with a trained actor to learn and practice more effective communication skills. Yet I am sure it is still not easy.

2   Robert M. Veatch, *A Theory of Medical Ethics,* Basic Books Inc., New York, 1981

3   Deborah Lupton, Doctors on the Medical Profession, *Sociology of Health and Illness,* 1997, 19(4) and Consumerism, Reflexivity and the Medical Encounter, *Social Science and Medicine,* 1997, 45(3). Interview with Norman Swan, *ABC Radio National Health Report,* December 1997

4   B. Williams, 'Patient Satisfaction: A valid concept?', *Social science and medicine,* 38(4), 1994

5   Martha Nussbaum, *The Fragility of Goodness, Luck and ethics in Greek tragedy and Philosophy.* Cambridge University Press, 1986

6   Lawrence Becker, 'Trust as Non-Cognitive Security about Motives', *Ethics,* 107, October 1996, pp. 43–61

7   Julia Medew, Health Editor, *Fairfax Media, The Age,* 12 April 2015

8   Julia Medew, *Fairfax Media,* 2 and 3 October 2015

9   Ken Lay, *Fairfax Media,* 11 March 2015

10 Nussbaum Martha, from *Take My Advice: Letters to the next generation from people who know a thing or two,* ed. James L Harmon, Simon and Schuster, New York, 2002

11 Carol-Anne Moulton, *Surgical News,* RACS, August 2014

12 Plato, *The Last days of Socrates, Phaedo,* 89d–90a, Tr. Christopher Rowe, Penguin Classics, 2010

13 Hegel, *The Philosophy of Right,* from *The Hegel Reader,* Ethical Life, ed. Stephen Hulgate, Blackwell, 1998

14 Richard Holton, 'Deciding to Trust, Coming to Believe', *Australasian Journal of Philosophy,* Vol. 72, March 1994

15 P.F. Strawson, *Freedom and Resentment,* Methuen London, 1974

16 Karen Jones, 'Trust as an Affective Attitude', *Ethics,* 107, October 1996

17 Philip Pettit, 'The Cunning of Trust', *Philosophy and Public Affairs,* 24, No. 3, Summer 1995

18 R.M. Hare, *The Language of Morals,* Clarendon Press, Oxford 1952, Chs. 1–3 & 11. See for discussion on using the word 'Ought'

19 Aristotle, *The Nicomachean Ethics*, Tr. David Ross, Oxford University Press, 1980

20 Michael Erant and Benedict du Boulay, University of Sussex, 2001, *Developing the Attributes of Medical Professional Judgement and Competence*. www.informatics. sussex.ac.uk/users/bend/doh. Accessed 24 June 2006

21 Atul Gawande, *Complications*, Profile Books Ltd., London, 2010

22 I have transposed and added to the example of the Sabre Tooth Cat given by Peter Singer in *How Are We to Live?*

23 Russell Hardin, 'Trusting persons, Trusting Institutions', in *The Strategy of Choice*, ed. Richard J. Zeckhauser, MIT Press Cambridge Mass, 1991

24 Russell Hardin, 'Trustworthiness', *Ethics*, 107, October 1996, pp. 26–42

25 Martin Hollis, *Trust within reason*, Cambridge University Press, Cambridge, 1998

26 Bertrand Russell, *The Problems of Philosophy*, Oxford University Press, 1997

27 Peter Singer, *How Are We to Live? Ethics in an Age of Self Interest*, Text Publishing, Melbourne, 1993

28 David Hume, *A Treatise of Human Nature*, Penguin Books, England, 1984

29 Robert Axelrod, *The Evolution of Cooperation*, Basic Books, New York, 1984, quoted in *Ethics*, ed. Peter Singer, 1994

30 Ernst Fehr, *On the Economics and Biology of Trust*, University of Zurich and IZA

31 Annette Baier, *Moral Prejudices, Essays on Ethics*, Harvard University Press, 1994

32 Bruno Malinowsky, *Argonauts of The Western Pacific*, Routledge and Kegan Paul (London 1922), in *Ethics*, ed. Peter Singer, Oxford University Press, 1994

33 Ann Daniel, *Scapegoats for a Profession, Uncovering Procedural Injustice*, Overseas Publishers Association, Amsterdam, 1998

34 Robert Trivers, 'The Evolution of Reciprocal Altruism', *Social Evolution*, Benjamin Cummings Publishing Company, California 1985, *Ethics*, ed. Peter Singer

35 *Tarasoff v. Regents of the University of California*, California Supreme Court, 17 California Reports. 3D Series, 425, 1 July 1976. See Tom L. Beauchamp & James F. Childress, *Principles of Biomedical Ethics*, third. ed. Oxford University Press, 1989

36 Ian N. Olver, Susan J. Turrell, N.A. Olszewski and Kristyn J. Wilson, 'Impact of an information and consent form on patients having chemotherapy', *The Medical Journal of Australia*, Vol. 162, 16 January 1995, pp. 80–3

37 J. Simes et. al., 'A randomised comparison of informed consent procedures in clinical trials', *British Medical Journal*, Vol. 294, 1986, pp. 1065–8

38 D. McCormack, D. Evoy, D. Mulcahy and M. Walsh, 'An evaluation of patients' comprehension of orthopaedic terminology: implications for informed consent', *Journal of The Royal College of Surgeons of Edinburgh*, February 1997, Vol. 42, No. 1, pp. 33–5

39 Neil C. Manson and Onora O'Neill, *Rethinking Informed Consent in Bioethics*,

Cambridge University Press, 2007

40 Merrilyn Walton, *The Trouble with Medicine, Preserving the trust with patients and doctors*, Allan and Unwin Australia, 1998

41 Francis Fukuyama, *Trust, The Social Virtues and The Creation of Prosperity*, Penguin Books, United Kingdom, 1995

42 Mason C.J., Brennan J., Dawson J., Toohy J., Gaudron M., McHugh J.J., *High Court of Australia: Christopher Rogers v. Marie Lynette Whitaker*, 1992, p. 790

43 Robert Veatch, 'Is Trust of Professionals a Coherent Concept in Ethics?' in *Trust and The Professions, Philosophical and Cultural Aspects*, ed. Edmond D. Pellegrino, Robert M. Veatch, John P. Langan, Georgetown University Press. Washington D.C., 1991

44 Immanuel Kant, *Foundations of the Metaphysics of Morals*, Macmillan, 1990

45 Christine M. Korsgaard, The Right to Lie: Kant on Dealing with Evil, *Philosophy and Public Affairs*, 1986, 15, pp. 329–32

46 Immanuel Kant, *The Metaphysical Principles of Virtue*, quoted by Korsgaard

47 Immanuel Kant, *Critique of Pure Reason*, quoted by Korsgaard

48 Robert Young, *Personal Autonomy: Beyond negative and Positive Liberty*, Croom Helm, London, 1986

49 Justin Oakley, 'Altruistic Surrogacy and Informed Consent', *Bioethics*, 6, No. 4, October 1992, pp. 269–87

50 Markus Freitag & Richard Traunmuller, Spheres of trust: An empirical analysis of the foundations of particularised and generalised trust, *European Journal of Political Research*, 2009, 48: 782–803, 849

51 Patrick Sturgis et. al., A Genetic Basis for Trust? *Polit Behav*, 2010, 32: 205–30

52 Constance A. Flanagan and Michael Stout, Developmental Patterns of Social Trust Between Early and Late Adolescence: Age and School Climate Effects, *Journal of Research on Adolescence*, 2010, 20(3), 748–73

53 Ebstein R.P., Israel S., Chew S.H., Zhong S., Knafol A., (2010), Genetics of Human Social Behaviour, *Neuron*

54 Zak, Paul J., The physiology of moral sentiments, *Journal of Economic Behavior and Organisation*, January 2011, pp. 53–65

55 Daniel Kahneman, 2011, *Thinking, Fast and Slow*, Penguin Books

56 Kuchinskas Susan, 2009, *The Chemistry of Connection*, New Harbinger Productions

57 Kogana Aleksandr, Laura R. Saslowb, Emily A. Impetta, Christopher Oveisc, Dacher Keltnerd, and Sarina Rodrigues Saturne, Thin-slicing study of the oxytocin receptor (OXTR)gene and the evaluation and expression of the prosocial disposition, *PNAS*, 29 November 2011, Vol. 108, No. 48

58 M. Stirrat and D.I. Perrett, Valid Facial Cues to Cooperation and Trust: Male

Facial Width and Trustworthiness, *Psychological Science*, 2010, 21: 349

59   Leslie J. Seltzer, Toni E. Ziegler and Seth D. Pollak, Social vocalizations can release oxytocin in humans, *Proc. R. Soc. B*, 2010, 277, 2661–6

60   Gottman John M., *The Science of Trust, Emotional Attunement for Couples*, W.W. Norton & Company, 2011

61   Di Pellegrino et. al., Understanding motor events: a neurophysiological study, *Experimental Brain Research*, 91, 176–80

62   *Medical Practitioners Board of Victoria, Annual Report*, 1995

63   Sissela Bok, *Lying: Moral Choice in Public and Private Life*, Pantheon Books, New York, 1978

64   Immanuel Kant, *The Foundations of the Metaphysics of Morals*, second ed. Lewis White Beck Translation, MacMillan, New York 1990 and *On a Supposed Right to Lie from Altruistic Motives*, appendix to Sissela Bok, *Lying*

65   Judith N. Shklar, 'The ambiguities of betrayal', *Ordinary Vices*, Harvard University Press Cambridge, 1984

66   Estlle Davison-Crews, 'Females in the Workplace, Acknowledging, Preventing Betrayal', *AORN Journal*, April 1990, Vol. 51, No. 4, pp. 1028–34

67   Tara Roth Madden, 'Woman vs. Woman: The Uncivil Business War', New York City, *AMACOM*, 1987

68   Charles Eccles-Smith and Justin Oakley, 'Informed Consent and Coronary by-pass Surgery', *Modern Medicine of Australia*, 1992, 35(9), pp. 98–104

69   Benjamin N. Cardozo 'Every human being of adult years and sound mind has a right to determine what shall be done with his own body.' *Schloendorff v. New York Hospital*, 211 N.Y., 1914

70   David Macintosh, 'Deceiving our patients', *Modern Medicine of Australia*, November 1993, pp. 58–60

71   'I will not abuse my position to indulge in sexual contacts with the bodies of women or of men, whether they be freemen or slaves'. *Hippocratic Writings*, ed. G.E.R. Lloyd, Trans. J. Chadwick and W. N. Mann, Penguin Classics, London, 1983, p. 67

72   Sheldon H. Kerdner, 'Sex and the Physician Patient Relationship', *American Journal of Psychiatry*, 131, October 74, pp. 134–6

73   Andrew L. Hyams, 'Expert Psychiatric Evidence in Sexual Misconduct Cases before State Medical Boards', *American Journal of Law and Medicine*, Vol. XVIII, No. 3, 1992, pp. 191–2

74   Ellen T. Luepker,' Sexual Exploitation of Clients by Therapists: Parallels with Parent Child Incest', in *Psychotherapists Sexual Involvement with Clients*: ed. Schoener Gary R. et. al., 1989

75   For a more complete analysis of sexual misconduct and trust, including Freud's views, see Merrilyn Walton, *The Trouble with Medicine, preserving the trust with*

patients and doctors, Allan and Unwin Australia, 1998, Ch. 4

76 Barry R. Furrow. 'Quality Control in Health Care', *The Journal of Law, Medicine and Ethics*, Vol. 21, No. 2, 1993, pp. 173–92

77 Yorker B.C. et al., Serial Murder by Healthcare Professionals, *J Forensic Science,* 2006 November, 51(6): 1362–71

78 Guthrie B. et al, Routine mortality monitoring for detecting mas murder in UK general practice: test of effectiveness using modelling. *Br J Gen Practice*, 2008 May, 58(550): 311–7

79 Richard Baker, Making haste slowly: the response to the Shipman enquiry? Editorial, *Br J Gen Practice*, 2008 May, 58(550)

80 Steve Clarke and Justin Oakley, *Informed Consent and Clinical Accountability: The Ethics of Report cards on Surgeon Performance*, 2007, Cambridge University Press

81 Geoffrey Davies. Ensuring the continuing competence of surgeons: a bridge too far, a sacred cow or burying your head in the sand. *ANZ J Surg.*, 2014 September, 84(9): 609–11

82 Bernard Barber, *The Logic and Limits of Trust*, Rutgers University Press New Jersey, 1983. See also Edmund D. Pellegrino & David C. Thomasma, *The Virtues in Medical Practice*, Oxford University Press, New York, 1993

83 High Court of Australia 156ALR517

84 Niklas Luhmann, *Trust and Power*, John Wiley and Sons, Pittman Press, Avon, 1979

85 Harold Garfinkel, *Studies in Ethnomethodology*, Englewood Cliffs, N.J. Prentice Hall, 1967

86 Ruth B. Purtilo & Christine K. Kassel, *Ethical Dimensions in The Health Professions*, W.B. Saunders, 1981

87 Edmond D. Pellegrino & David C. Thomasma, *Helping and Healing: Religious Commitment in Health Care*, Georgetown University Press, Washington, 1997

88 Foucault, *The Birth of The Clinic, The Foucault Reader,* ed. P. Rabinow, Harnondsworth, Penguin Books, 1994

89 John Locke, *Essays on the Law of Nature* (1663), Chapter 8. 'Is Every Man's Interest the Basis of the Law of Nature? No', ed. W. Von Leyden, Oxford Clarendon Press, 1974

90 John Dunn, *Locke*, Past Masters, Oxford University Press, 1984

91 *Hegel's Philosophy of Right*, Tr. T. N. Knox, Oxford University Press, 1967

92 Frank Costigan Q.C., 'Corruption at the End of the Twentieth Century', *Melbourne University Magazine*, Spring 1999, p. 12

93 John Rawls, 'Outline of a decision procedure for ethics', *Philosophical Review*, 60(2) 1951, pp. 177–97

94 *Herald Sun*, 14 October 1993, p. 23 (reprinted from the *Daily Mail*)

95 Lawrence A. Blum, 'Gilligan and Kohlberg: Implications for Moral Theory', *Ethics*, 98, April 1998

96 P.J. van der Mass et. al., 'Euthanasia and other medical decisions concerning the end of life', *The Lancet*, 338, September 14, 1991

97 Lawrence A. Blum, 'Vocation, Friendship, and Community: Limitations of the Personal-Impersonal Framework, from Identity, Character, and Morality', *Essays in Moral Psychology*, ed. Owen Flannigan and A.O. Rorty, Cambridge MIT Press, 1990

98 Herbert Kohl, *Growing Minds: On Becoming a Teacher*, Harper and Row, New York, 1984

99 Aristotle, *The Art of Rhetoric*, Tr. H.C. Lawson-Tancred, Penguin Books, 1991

100 Aristotle, *De Anima*, Tr. H.C. Lawson-Tancred, Penguin Books, 1986

101 Jean Decety et al., *Neuroimage*, 14 January 2010

102 Michael Stocker & Elizabeth Hedgeman, *Valuing Emotions*, Cambridge Studies in Philosophy, Cambridge University Press, 1996

103 Neil Armfield, *Company B Belvoir St. production of Hamlet, Melbourne Theatre Company*, programme notes, 1995

104 Judith N. Shklar, 'The ambiguities of betrayal', *Ordinary Vices*, Harvard University Press, Cambridge, 1984

105 Thomas Hobbes, *Leviathan* ed. John Planenatz, Fontana Books, 1974

106 Young, Iris Marion, *Justice and the Politics of Difference*, Princeton University Press, 1990

107 Plato, *Alcibiades, 1 132C–133B*

108 Peter Singer, *Hegel*, Oxford University Press, 1983

109 J.D. Wallace, *Virtues and Vices*, Ithaca Cornell University Press, 1978

110 L.E. Mitchell, (2001) The importance of being trusted, *Boston University Law Review*, 81, 591–657

111 *Les Miserable*, from the novel by Victor Hugo, music by Claude-Michel Schonberg, English lyrics by Herbert Krezmer

112 Raymond Chandler, *The Big Sleep*, Penguin books, 1970

113 We act as though concepts like goodness or justice have real substance in themselves. For a discussion on how ethical thought and action appears to be objectively based even if this appearance is in error see J. L. Mackie, *Ethics, Inventing Right and Wrong*, Penguin London, 1977, Ch. 1

114 Aristotle, *The Politics*, Tr. T. A. Sinclair, Penguin Books, 1992

115 Lao Tzu. I cannot remember where I saw this translation. It is phrased slightly differently in the *Tao Te Ching*, Tr. Man-Ho Kwok, Martin Palmer & Jay Ramsey, Element Classic Editions, Element Books Ltd., Dorset, 1994

116 Thucydides, *History of the Peloponnesian War*, Tr. Benjamin Jowett, Vol. 1, quoted by Peter Johnson in *Frames of Deceit*, Cambridge University Press, 1993

117 Niccolo Machiavelli, *The Prince*, Penguin Classics, 1961

118 Niccolo Machiavelli, *The Prince and The Discourses*, The Modern Library, New York, 1950

119 Salman Rushdie, *The Moor's Last Sigh*, Jonathan Cape, London, 1995

120 Adam Smith, *The Theory of Moral Sentiments*, Prometheus Books, New York, 2000

121 Plato, *The Republic*, Penguin, 1973

122 J.S. Mill, *Utilitarianism, On Liberty, and Considerations on Representative Government*, ed. H.B. Acton, J.M. Dent & Sons Ltd., 1972

123 Max Charlesworth, *Bioethics in a Liberal Society*, Cambridge University Press, 1993

124 W.D. Ross, *The Right and the Good*, Oxford University Press, 1930

125 Gilligan Carol, *In a Different Voice: Psychological Theory and Women's Development*, Harvard University Press, 1992

126 I owe the basis of this idea to Iris Young

127 American Psychological Association, (2006). *Forgiveness: A Sampling of Research Results*. Washington, DC: Office of International Affairs. Reprinted, 2008

128 Susan Whitbourne, *Live Longer by Practising Forgiveness* www.psychologytoday.com/blog/fulfilment-any-age/201301/live-longer-practicing-forgiveness, accessed 23 February 2015

129 Jill Stark, *Fairfax Media, The Age*, 12 April 2015

130 Hannah Arendt, *The Human Condition*, The University of Chicago Press, 1998

131 Judith Orloff, *Emotional Freedom: Liberate Yourself from Negative Emotions and Transform Your Life*, Harmony Books, New York, 2013

132 Brene Brown, TED.com, recorded June 2010, accessed 7 August 2013

133 Peter Johnson, *Frames of Deceit*, Cambridge University Press, 1993

Acknowledgments

Peter Singer and Helga Kuhse for establishing the Master's degree in Bioethics at Monash University and inspiring me to further study and being responsible for a gratifying change in my career.

Justin Oakley for years of supervising my Ph.D. thesis and teaching me so much. At times it is not possible for me to separate my ideas from his, such has been his influence. My sub-title honours his book *Morality and the Emotions*.

Nick Walker for seeing things other publishers did not and making me shed tears of relief and gratitude.

Amelia Walker for a striking cover design.

Beverley Macintosh for helping me begin the journey.

Belinda Pearson for constant support and help in so many ways.

Anne Bolch of *A Story to Tell* for a very professional job of editing and much good advice.

Lee Sandwith of *DONE. TOTAL BUSINESS SOLUTIONS* for excellent and enthusiastic marketing.

Danielle McClurg of Creative Fold Design for a great website.

Kate Morris for some important suggestions in making the book more readable.

Jackie Hill and Maureen Bell for helping to open my eyes during a delicious and entertaining dinner party.

Marilyn McDonald for delighting, enlightening and forgiving me in just once sentence.

Colette Johnson and Debra Norris for many hours of listening and typing.

Elizabeth Smith and Ian Macintosh for critical editing in the earlier stages and who at last had some revenge for the sometimes harsh literary criticisms of their loving father.

Sarndra Mitting for sparking my resolve to write this book and some vital contributions.

Helen Henderson for encouragement, indexing and editing.

The thousands of patients who have helped me. I hope I have returned the favour more often than not.

My many surgical and medical colleagues. I have always been proud to stand amongst them.

Index

Stirrat, M. 101, 200
Stout, Michael 94, 200
Stratford, Angela 140, 141
Sturgis, Patrick 93, 94, 95, 200
sympathy 30, 48, 49, 72, 90, 91, 95, 112, 183, 191, 195

Tan , Caroline 10
Tarasoff, Tatania 67
The Aeneid 159
The Big Sleep 170, 203
the Mean 48
The Merchant of Venice 177, 185
Thomasma, David 130, 202
Thucydides 173, 204
'Tit for Tat' 60, 61, 62, 63, 64, 180, 184, 190, 196
Tortilla Flat 168
total hip replacement 81, 86, 87, 175
Traunmuller, Michael 93, 200
Trivers, Robert 64, 199
trust *passim*; trustee 23, 24, 25, 26, 27, 29, 30, 40, 42, 43, 65, 99, 103, 115, 140, 147, 163–174, 181, 190, 191, 192, 195; truster 9, 23, 24, 25, 26, 30, 40, 41, 42, 43, 93, 99, 102, 108, 149, 167, 169, 171, 181, 191, 195; trustworthiness 2, 7, 14, 16, 17, 20, 22, 24, 25, 28, 29, 48, 52, 55, 56, 61, 62, 66, 89, 93, 99, 101, 102, 116, 132, 134, 135, 141, 144, 150, 155, 160, 161, 166, 167, 168, 169, 173, 174, 185, 187, 188, 190, 193, 195, 196, 197

uncertainty 2, 52, 53, 89, 153, 159, 192

United Bristol Health Care Trust 123
universalisation 82, 83

Valjean, Jean 168
values 7, 10, 22, 42, 54, 55, 65, 66, 67, 70, 75, 76, 78, 79, 89, 90, 106, 107, 109, 113, 126, 132, 135, 138, 139, 142, 143, 144, 146, 149, 150, 153, 160, 161, 164, 165, 166, 168, 169, 176, 178, 188, 193, 194
Van de Mass, P.J. 142, 203
Veatch, Robert 77, 78, 79, 198, 200
Virgil 159
virtues 40, 47, 48, 49, 50, 77, 78, 85, 111, 116, 117, 138, 142, 145, 146, 153, 161, 174, 190, 193, 194, 197
vocation 64, 116, 142, 143, 144, 151, 166, 168, 194, 195, 197
vulnerability 1, 2, 9, 41, 101, 131, 176, 184

Walter, Harold 163
Walton, Merrilyn 72

Yorker, B.C. 121, 202
Young, Iris 164, 203, 204
Young, Robert 84, 200

Zac, Paul 95, 96, 99, 100, 200

Printed in Australia
AUHW011137080319
309561AU00003B/11